GASTROENTER
IN PRIMARY C

Gastroenterology in Primary Care

An evidence-based guide to management

Edited by

Pali Hungin
MB BS MD FRCGP DRCOG
Professor, Centre for Health Studies, University of Durham
General Practitioner, Eaglescliffe, Stockton on Tees

Greg Rubin
MB ChB FRCGP
Senior Lecturer, University of Teesside
General Practitioner, Thornaby, Stockton on Tees

Foreword by Roger Jones

**Blackwell
Science**

© 2000 by
Blackwell Science Ltd
Editorial Offices:
Osney Mead, Oxford OX2 0EL
25 John Street, London WC1N 2BL
23 Ainslie Place, Edinburgh EH3 6AJ
350 Main Street, Malden
 MA 02148-5018, USA
54 University Street, Carlton
 Victoria 3053, Australia
10, rue Casimir Delavigne
 75006 Paris, France

Other Editorial Offices:
Blackwell Wissenschafts-Verlag GmbH
Kurfürstendamm 57
10707 Berlin, Germany

Blackwell Science KK
MG Kodenmacho Building
7–10 Kodenmacho Nihombashi
Chuo-ku, Tokyo 104, Japan

The right of the Author to be
identified as the Author of this Work
has been asserted in accordance
with the copyright, Designs and
Patents Act 1988.

First published 2000

Set by Graphicraft Limited, Hong Kong
Printed and bound in Great Britain
at the Alden Press Ltd, Oxford and
Northampton

The Blackwell Science logo is a
trade mark of Blackwell Science Ltd,
registered at the United Kingdom
Trade Marks Registry

DISTRIBUTORS

Marston Book Services Ltd
PO Box 269
Abingdon, Oxon OX14 4YN
(*Orders:* Tel: 01235 465500
         Fax: 01235 465555)

USA
Blackwell Science, Inc
Commerce Place
350 Main Street
Malden, MA 02148-5018
(*Orders:* Tel: 781 388 8250
         Fax: 781 388 8255)

Canada
Login Brothers Book Company
324 Saulteaux Cresent
Winnipeg, Manitoba R3J 3T2
(*Orders:* Tel: 204 837 2987)

Australia
Blackwell Science Pty Ltd
54 University Street
Carlton, Victoria 3053
(*Orders:* Tel: 3 9347 0300
         Fax: 3 9347 5001)

A catalogue record for this title
is available from the British Library

ISBN 0-632-04793-3

Library of Congress
Cataloging-in-publication Data

Gastroenterology in primary care: an
evidence-based guide to management/editors,
Pali Hungin, Greg Rubin.
      p. cm.
   Includes bibliographical references.
   ISBN 0-632-05191-4
   1 Gastrointestinal system—Diseases.
   2 Primary care (Medicine).   3 Evidence-
   based medicine.   I Hungin, Pali.
   II Rubin, Greg.
      [DNLM: 1 Gastrointestinal Diseases—
   diagnosis.   2 Gastrointestinal Diseases
   —therapy.   3 Evidence-Based Medicine.
   4 Primary Health Care.
   WI 141 G2573   2000]
   RC816.G37   2000
   616.3'3 21; aa05 10-27—dc99
                                    99-054485

For further information on
Blackwell Science, visit our website:
www.blackwell-science.com

Contents

List of contributors, vii

Foreword, ix

Preface, xi

1 Translating evidence into individual care, 1
   Anthony Roberts and Toby Lipman

2 Gastro-oesophageal reflux disease, 9
   Pali Hungin

3 Dyspepsia and *Helicobacter pylori*, 23
   Greg Rubin

4 Gastric cancer, 33
   Michael Bramble

5 Gallbladder and biliary problems, 39
   Pali Hungin

6 Liver problems, 45
   Michael Bramble

7 Acute and chronic pancreatitis, 57
   Michael Bramble

8 Irritable bowel syndrome, 61
   Robin Spiller

9 Coeliac disease and malabsorption problems, 73
   John Silcock

10 Inflammatory bowel disease, 81
   John Mansfield

11 Constipation, diarrhoea and minor anal disorders, 91
   Greg Rubin

12 Colorectal cancer, 99
   Rob Wilson

   Index, 105

List of contributors

Michael Bramble MD FRCP
Consultant Physician and Gastroenterologist, South Cleveland Hospital, Middlesborough
Honorary Professor, Centre for Health Studies, University of Durham

Pali Hungin MD FRCGP DRCOG
Professor, Centre for Health Studies, University of Durham
General Practitioner, Eaglescliffe, Stockton on Tees
Honorary Treasurer, Primary Care Society for Gastroenterology

Toby Lipman MRCGP
General Practitioner, Westerhope, Newcastle upon Tyne
NHSE Northern and Yorkshire Regional Research Training Fellow

John Mansfield MA MB BS MD MRCP
Consultant Gastroenterologist, Royal Victoria Infirmary, Newcastle upon Tyne
Senior Lecturer, University of Newcastle upon Tyne

Anthony Roberts BA MA CIM Diploma Marketing MSc
Honorary Research Fellow, Centre for Health Studies, University of Durham
Clinical Effectiveness Advisor, Primary Care Resource and Development Centre, Teesside

Greg Rubin MB BS FRCGP
Senior Lecturer, University of Teesside
General Practitioner, Thornaby, Stockton on Tees
Honorary Secretary, Primary Care Society for Gastroenterology

John Silcock MD FRCP
Consultant Gastroenterologist, South Cleveland Hospital, Middlesborough

Robin Spiller MA(Cantab) MSc(Lond) MB BChir MD(Cantab) FRCP
Reader in Gastroenterology, University Hospital, Nottingham

Rob Wilson MD FRCS
Consultant Surgeon, South Cleveland Hospital
Senior Lecturer, University of Newcastle upon Tyne

Foreword

Gastroenterology is important in general practice. Around 10% of consultations are related to digestive disorders and the costs of prescribing and hospital treatment of many gastrointestinal problems are substantial. Gastrointestinal illness has a significant negative impact on patients' quality of life and their ability to function at work and at home. Paradoxically the common gastrointestinal disorders, with the exception of colorectal cancer, rarely feature prominently in national and regional health strategies, so the publication of this book is a timely reminder to general practitioners, at a time of unprecedented organizational change in the National Health Service, of the significance of digestive diseases.

Digestive symptoms are extremely common in the general population. Well-conducted epidemiological surveys have demonstrated that around 40% of the adult population experience significant dyspepsia and gastro-oesophageal reflux symptoms every year, and that about one quarter of individuals report a symptom complex compatible with a clinical diagnosis of irritable bowel syndrome (IBS). Rectal bleeding is experienced by between 10% and 15% of people every year, many of whom have concomitant lower bowel symptoms. Yet only a minority of these people turn into patients and seek medical advice for their symptoms – around 25% for dyspepsia and IBS and 35% for rectal bleeding. The factors affecting the decision to consult a general practitioner include patients' perceptions of the significance and meaning of their symptoms, their fears of cancer or other serious disease, the severity of the symptoms themselves and the individual's psychological state. The first step in the management of these symptoms in primary care involves disentangling the physical presentation from the background mosaic of health beliefs, anxieties, learnt illness behaviour and socio-psychological dysfunction.

The task of the primary care physician has been characterized as 'marginalizing danger', while that of the specialist is to 'marginalize uncertainty'. Patients often present with a confusing array of symptoms, and a clinical diagnosis is often difficult to make on the basis of symptoms alone. On many occasions, the best we can do is to try to decide, using the evidence linking 'alarm symptoms' with serious organic disease, whether or not the patient requires urgent investigation, treatment or referral. Often this is difficult because the predictive values of individual symptoms and symptom complexes for a final, organic diagnosis are often low or unknown.

Diagnosis and management in primary care frequently employ time as a diagnostic tool; symptoms that may have been worrying at first may disappear, while other vague complaints may gradually form themselves into a more discernible syndrome for which appropriate measures can be taken. This means that many of our decisions about prescribing, investigation and referral are based on imperfect evidence—imperfect partly because of the partial stories offered to us by our patients, but also because of the relative paucity of well-conducted studies of the natural history of digestive disorders in primary care. Many of the recommendations that form the basis of guidelines, protocols and management plans are derived from studies carried out in secondary care settings, which may not be applicable to patients seen in general practice.

It follows that, as well as providing a guide to the existing evidence, a book like this also highlights areas of ignorance, where the evidence is simply not available. The need for more research in primary care is evident from reading the chapters in this book, and the questions raised by an unsuccessful search for evidence on which to base best practice amount to a research agenda in primary care gastroenterology.

In the new world of primary care groups (PCGs), clinical governance, guidelines, the National Institute for Clinical Excellence and the National Electronic Library for Health, we are engaged on a search for the evidence which will ensure that our patients receive the best possible care, consonant with the resources available within the health service. The individual general practitioner consulting this book will find a useful resumé of the important topics in gastroenterology in primary care and practical recommendations directed towards best practice. Clinical governance leads in PCGs will, similarly, find a clear account of priorities for resource allocation in gastrointestinal disorders and, where it is available, the evidence on which to base standards of care. Anyone in search of algorithmic certainties is likely to be disappointed. Just as clinical freedom was described as 'at best a cloak for ignorance and at worst an excuse for quackery', so the current vogue for protocol-driven care is in danger of concealing gaps in knowledge, suppressing curiosity and subordinating the doctor–patient relationship to a series of decision nodes. An understanding of each patient's individual circumstances, their hopes, fears and expectations, and the limitations of much current 'evidence' lies at the heart of effective primary care.

Roger Jones
Wolfson Professor of General Practice
Guy's, King's and St Thomas' School of Medicine, London

Preface

'The greater the ignorance the greater the dogmatism.'
William Osler

Much of how we practise is based on what has been learnt through the traditions of medicine, the long apprenticeship every doctor serves and our personal experiences. Perhaps the most enduring quality of the good clinician is the readiness to keep an open mind and to learn continuously. Evidence-based medicine, a concept not necessarily wrought of clinicians themselves, is having a profound effect on the way the quality and validity of the clinical process are judged.

Not everything is evidence based: in those fields where meta-analyses of randomized controlled trials abound, it is relatively easy to advise on the 'correct' course of action. Some specialities are better suited to this approach. Many problems in gastroenterology are closely related to health behaviour and human problems and are, not surprisingly, relatively devoid of the sort of evidence that renders certainty based on research. Much current gastroenterological practice is based on reasoning rather than tested reasons. Whereas there are any number of clinical trials involving drugs these are often secondary care based and rarely compare different regimens. Placebo response rates are high—up to 50% in patients with irritable bowel syndrome—and many established treatments, including the use of dietary fibre, have been based on vogue rather than clear-cut 'evidence'.

A book like this, if based entirely on hard 'evidence' derived from primary care, would have been very thin indeed and would have missed the point of trying to collate robust approaches for the management of problems in general practice. No apology is offered for the paucity of comparison charts and 'numbers needed to treat'; in most cases such data simply do not exist. The authors have provided current advice within the brief of being as evidence based as possible. The aim of this book is to assist the general practitioner and the patient in the clinical setting.

Pali Hungin
Greg Rubin

1 Translating evidence into individual care

Anthony Roberts and Toby Lipman

Key Points

- Evidence-based gastroenterology is the conscientious, explicit and judicious use of current best evidence in making decisions about the care of individual patients with problems of the digestive tract. This means integrating individual clinical expertise with the best available external clinical evidence from systematic research.
- Clinical expertise is: '... the proficiency and judgement acquired through clinical experience and practice. Increased expertise is reflected in many ways, but especially in more effective and efficient diagnosis and in the more thoughtful identification and compassionate use of individual patients' predicaments, rights and preferences in making clinical decisions about their care' [1].

Background

During the last decade, discussion of evidence-based medicine (EBM) has snowballed. A Medline search on the term 'evidence-based medicine' retrieved 86 articles between 1991 and 1995, but over 1700 between 1996 and 1999. Much of the literature describes the methodology and process of EBM [2–5] but there has also been intense debate both for and against it [6–10].

Although it originated in general medicine, the principles of EBM can be applied in any field of health care as evidence-based practice, evidence-based mental health, evidence-based health policy and so on. A definition of evidence-based gastroenterology, adapted from a classic definition of evidence-based medicine [1], is given in the key points box.

That the diagnosis and treatment of gastroenterological conditions should be based upon the best current scientific evidence is, on the face

1

of it, a truism, so clinicians, patients, policy makers and the general public may be forgiven for wondering why EBM excites such controversy. Sackett and colleagues originally described how to integrate clinical epidemiology and critical appraisal of research findings into routine clinical practice, together with more efficient ways of keeping up to date, and later applied the label 'evidence-based medicine' to their methods [11]. Evidence-based medicine is only one of a number of possible responses to the problems of widespread variations in clinical practice, the continuing use of ineffective or dangerous interventions, and unacceptable delays between the availability of research evidence and its routine implementation [12]. These responses include, especially, the use of clinical guidelines [13] and audit [14].

What is 'evidence'?

It is not so much the idea that evidence should be used that is controversial, but which evidence? By what process? On whose authority? Traditionally, medicine is perceived as a relatively fixed body of knowledge which students must master before being admitted to the profession. This knowledge is 'owned' and given validity by the authority of senior members of the profession. Doctors expect (and are expected) to know which treatment to give or which investigation to order for which disease. They are taught from the start that ignorance, or the appearance of ignorance, is unacceptable, and that, as is also the position in law, correct management is what a body of experts says it is. The history of medicine is littered with examples of experts in senior positions promoting ineffective interventions or being slow to adopt effective ones.* In the nineteenth century it took a generation for the profession to accept and act upon the observations of Semelweiss and Wendell Holmes that hand washing between examining patients dramatically reduced mortality from puerperal sepsis [15]. In the 1960s, a former president of the American College of Surgeons promoted the use of gastric freezing, in which balloons filled with coolant at a temperature of $-10°C$ were inserted into the stomachs of patients with peptic ulcer to reduce gastric acid secretion. This was enthusiastically taken up by many other surgeons on the basis of their senior colleague's authority,

---

* '. . . to base your treatment of commonly encountered problems on the advice of some "expert" who publishes treatment recommendations but no supporting evidence puts you on a par with the barefoot doctor. After all, it was these same experts who advocated turpentine stopes and leeches' [11].

but ultimately abandoned when a randomized controlled trial demonstrated no benefit nearly 10 years later [11].

Authority is not only no guarantee of sound advice, but a dangerously slow mechanism by which to incorporate advances in scientific knowledge into practice. As the pace of advance in gastroenterology continues to increase, the volume of published research militates against practising clinicians keeping up to date. They need an efficient method for finding and using the research literature. The key advantages of evidence-based gastroenterology are that it offers efficiency in identifying relevant evidence and facilitates greater explicitness in the evaluation of new research in terms of validity, clinical usefulness and local applicability.

Evidence-based medicine: imposition of management rules?

Evidence-based medicine raises fears that it will mean the imposition of clinical management rules which must be adhered to unthinkingly. On the contrary, exponents of EBM emphasize that research evidence cannot be applied mechanistically, but should be integrated with clinical expertise (see the key points box at the beginning of the chapter). Moreover, far from blind obedience to imposed standards, EBM requires that clinicians continually question their practice and, above all, actively seek out areas of uncertainty in their knowledge and understanding. This contradicts the traditional assumptions of authority-based medicine because the explicit recognition of ignorance now becomes a virtue rather than a failing, and is the driving force behind the formulation of answerable questions.

Evidence-based medicine: new skills needed

These changes in attitude and behaviour are profound, and the new skills and techniques that must be acquired are formidable. Evidence-based medicine constitutes a paradigm shift in medical practice, a revolutionary change in view made necessary by the inability of the old approach (authority- or tradition-based medicine) to meet the demands of modern practice [16,17]. This leads to suggestions that EBM is promulgated by academics safely cloistered in ivory towers. However, audits have shown that the majority of inpatients treated within units striving to provide evidence-based care do indeed receive evidence-based interventions. Furthermore, the NHS reforms of 1997

1

require, as part of clinical governance (the requirement of NHS health care organizations to be accountable for the quality of the clinical care they deliver) that 'a quality organization will ensure that evidence-based practice is in day to day use with the infrastructure to support it' [18].

Objections to evidence-based medicine

A common criticism is that EBM largely relies on randomized controlled trials (RCTs) (or systematic reviews and meta-analyses of such trials). When the central question concerns the balance of good and harm produced by a therapy, the most reliable (or least biased) way of researching the question is by using RCTs or meta-analyses. However, it must be recognized that, while questions about therapies are important, they are not the only questions that need answers in clinical practice. Questions may arise concerning the accuracy of diagnostic tests, the usefulness of prognostic markers, the acceptability of treatments to patients and the assessment of health-care needs. Methodologies should be governed by the questions to which answers are sought [19].

The emphasis on the quantitative aspects of EBM has led to anxieties that the art of medicine is endangered by an over-emphasis on biomedical science. Evidence-based medicine is also criticized for being reductionist and distanced from problems and decisions for the individual patient [20,21]. However, the proponents of EBM, like Greenhalgh, point out that questions should, where appropriate, be answered in qualitative as well as quantitative terms. Current developments in the field of EBM are exploring the need to reconcile individual human situations, often beset with complex clinical and personal needs, with the probabilistic focus of most clinical research [22,23].

Evidence-based medicine: a means of reducing costs and access to care?

Some doctors may fear that EBM could be used to control the costs of health care by reducing access. However, in EBM the focus should remain the individual patient and the doctor seeking to provide the best care (in terms of the quantity and quality of life) may well contribute to raising costs. None the less, clinicians using EBM can create strategies that balance benefits to individual patients and to society at large. This can be done, for example, by the abandonment of ineffective procedures, using less expensive but proven interventions and adopting newer interventions that reduce costs in the longer run. Maynard has pointed out the potential conflict between 'treatment decisions . . . dominated by clinicians and the individual-patient ethic of effectiveness, rather than by the population-health ethic of efficiency' [24,25]. Evidence of clinical effectiveness is not in itself sufficient to answer questions about economic efficiency. These require economic evaluations, which add a further important dimension to evidence-based health care. For example, a systematic review of the clinical effectiveness of treatments for gastro-oesophageal reflux disease can be used as the basis of a cost-effectiveness analysis of those treatments [26,27]. Economic evaluations can be critically appraised for validity and applicability in the same way as any other study and used to inform decision making.

Practising evidence-based medicine

While caring for patients, the need for information about diagnosis, treatment and prognosis continually arises. Medical science too is in a state of continuous change, necessitating a questioning attitude to current practice. Evidence-based medicine defines five steps to meet these needs for information (Table 1.1) [3].

A good starting point for an EBM approach is to ask of any clinical action 'what am I likely to achieve by this intervention?' The 'intervention' might be a question ('when did your heartburn start?'), physical examination (palpating the epigastrium), prescribing a drug (a bottle of antacid) or ordering a test (upper gastrointestinal endoscopy) [3]. Searching skills are important and clinicians increasingly require access to databases such as Medline, the Cochrane Library and the Internet. Integration of information technology into the practice setting is a

Table 1.1 Steps in meeting a need for information.

1 Converting the information need into answerable questions
2 Tracking down the best available research evidence with maximum efficiency
3 Critically appraising the evidence for its validity (closeness to the truth) and importance (its clinical applicability)
4 Estimating, using clinical expertise, the risks and responses of individual patients and their values and preferences, integrating these with the appraised evidence and applying the result in clinical practice
5 Evaluating performance to see whether the outcomes for patients are consistent with the expected outcomes predicted in this process

1

requisite requirement for the enthusiastic EBM practitioner [28]. Critical appraisal skills enable the clinician to make the most use of existing research, by assessing its validity, applicability and clinical importance in the form of quantification of effect sizes (e.g. absolute and relative risk reductions and numbers needed to treat). This can be done using critical appraisal checklists, of which excellent examples are given by Sackett [3] and Greenhalgh [5]. Evaluating performance includes clinical audit and assessing the educational process itself. This process integrates learning with clinical care and is perhaps best seen as an addition to, rather than a replacement for, the traditional clinical methods of history and examination. What it does replace is potentially passive and ineffective education methods (such as lectures by experts) with active and more effective methods such as small group learning [29–31].

It is unrealistic to expect clinicians, especially in general practice, with its severe time constraints, to go through this process in full with every patient they see, any more than they would do a complete history and physical examination in every consultation. However, they need to understand the concepts and application of EBM when appropriate, just as they need to know how and when to examine a particular part of the body. Fortunately, publications such as *Evidence-Based Medicine* and databases such as the Cochrane Library and Best Evidence provide pre-appraised evidence which, if the clinician understands the process of EBM, can often be used to inform decisions in practice without the need to tackle the full texts of original research papers. In addition, publications such as the present volume offer summaries of current evidence in specific clinical areas.

Conclusions

Evidence-based medicine combines a number of techniques and skills into a structured process which is designed to identify the need for information about health-care management, efficiently search for that information, critically appraise it and use it in clinical practice. It does not replace, but adds to, established clinical skills by integrating continuing education with patient care. Clinicians will need support to acquire the necessary expertise and extensive infrastructure to use it, including routine access to electronic information sources and libraries. Identifying gaps in personal knowledge as the trigger for self-directed searches for information is a valuable professional attribute. This process enhances the clinician's ability not only to identify the most effective interventions, but, because the process starts with real life patients' individual clinical problems, to work more effectively with them in joint decision making.

References

1 Sackett DL, Rosenberg WM, Gray JA, Haynes RB, Richardson WS. Evidence based medicine: what it is and what it isn't [editorial] [see comments]. *BMJ* 1996; **312** (7023): 71–2.

2 Rosenberg W, Donald A. Evidence based medicine: an approach to clinical problem-solving [see comments]. *BMJ* 1995; **310** (6987): 1122–6.

3 Sackett DL, Richardson WS, Rosenberg W, Haynes RB. *Evidence-based Medicine: How to Practice and Teach EBM.* London: Churchill Livingstone, 1997.

4 Sackett DL, Straus SE. Finding and applying evidence during clinical rounds: the 'evidence cart' [see comments]. *JAMA* 1998; **280** (15): 1336–8.

5 Greenhalgh T. How to read a paper. *The Basics of Evidence-Based Medicine.* London: BMJ Publishing Group, 1997.

6 Rosenberg WM, Sackett DL. On the need for evidence-based medicine. *Therapie* 1996; **51** (3): 212–17.

7 Charlton BG, Miles A. The rise and fall of EBM. *Q J Med* 1998; **91** (5): 371–4.

8 Marshall T. Evidence-based medicine [letter; comment]. *Lancet* 1995; **346** (8983): 1171–2.

9 Naylor CD. Grey zones of clinical practice: some limits to evidence-based medicine. *Lancet* 1995; **345** (8953): 840–2.

10 Leggett JM. Medical scientism: good practice or fatal error? *J R Soc Med* 1997; **90** (2): 97–101.

11 Sackett DL, Haynes RB, Guyatt GH, Tugwell P. *Clinical Epidemiology: A Basic Science for Clinical Medicine,* 2nd edn, p. 193. Boston: Little, Brown and Company, 1991.

12 Haines A, Jones R. Implementing findings of research [see comments]. *BMJ* 1994: **308** (6942): 1488–92.

13 Grimshaw J, Eccles M, Russell I. Developing clinically valid practice guidelines. *J Evaluation Clin Prac* 1995; **1** (1): 37–48.

14 Houghton G. From audit to effectiveness: an historical evaluation of the changing role of Medical Audit Advisory Groups. *J Evaluation Clin Prac* 1997; **3** (4): 245–53.

15 Lloyd WEB. *A Hundred Years of Medicine,* 2nd edn. London: Duckworth, 1968.

16 Anonymous. Evidence-based medicine. A new approach to teaching the practice of medicine. Evidence-Based Medicine Working Group [see comments]. *JAMA* 1992; **268** (17): 2420–5.

17 Kuhn TS. *The Structure of Scientific Revolutions.* Chicago: University of Chicago Press, 1970.

18 Secretary of State for Health. The new NHS, modern, dependable. London: HMSO, 1997.

19 Sackett DL, Wennberg JE. Choosing the best research design for each question [editorial]. *BMJ* 1997; **315** (7123): 1636.

20 Sweeney K. How can evidence-based medicine help patients in general practice? [Editorial] *Family Prac* 1996; **13** (6): 489–90.

1

21 Jacobson LD, Edwards AG, Granier SK, Butler CC. Evidence-based medicine and general practice [see comments]. *Br J General Prac* 1997; **47** (420): 449–52.

22 Greenhalgh T. Is my practice evidence-based? [Editorial] *BMJ* 1996; **313** (7063): 957–8.

23 Greenhalgh T. Narrative based medicine: narrative based medicine in an evidence based world. *BMJ* 1999; **318** (7179): 323–5.

24 Maynard A. Evidence-based medicine: an incomplete method for informing treatment choices [see comments]. *Lancet* 1997; **349** (9045): 126–8.

25 Maynard A. Evidence-based medicine. Cost effectiveness and equity are ignored [letter; comment]. *BMJ* 1996; **313** (7050): 170–1.

26 Moore RA, Wiffen P, McQuay HJ, Phillips C. Reflux oesophagitis: quantitative systematic review of the evidence of effectiveness of proton pump inhibitors and histamine antagonists. Vol 4, Issue no. 36. Bandolier Internet Publications, 1997 (http://www.jr2.ox.ac.uk/Bandolier).

27 Phillips C, Moore A. Trial and error – an expensive luxury: economic analysis of effectiveness of proton pump inhibitors and histamine antagonists in treating reflux disease. *Br J Med Economics* 1997; **11**: 55–63.

28 Purves IN. Facing future challenges in general practice: a clinical method with computer support. *Family Prac* 1996; **13** (6): 536–43.

29 Onion CW, Bartzokas CA. Changing attitudes to infection management in primary care: a controlled trial of active versus passive guideline implementation strategies. *Family Prac* 1998; **15** (2): 99–104.

30 van Leeuwen YD, Mol SS, Pollemans MC, Drop MJ, Grol R, van der Vleuten CP. Change in knowledge of general practitioners during their professional careers. *Family Prac* 1995; **12** (3): 313–17.

31 Rogers S. Evidence-based learning for general practice [letter; comment]. *Br J General Prac* 1997; **47** (414): 52–3.

2 Gastro-oesophageal reflux disease

Pali Hungin

Key Points

- Gastro-oesophageal reflux disease is experienced by 40% of the population in a 6-month period.
- Heartburn and regurgitation as dominant symptoms have a high level of diagnostic specificity.
- Investigate by gastroscopy if alarm symptoms present, new onset at age over 45 or poor response to empirical treatment.

What causes gastro-oesophageal reflux disease?

The cause of gastro-oesophageal reflux disease (GORD) is thought to be repeated reflux of gastric acid onto the oesophageal mucosa [1]. The chief factors contributing are: (i) reduced lower oesophageal sphincter pressure, leading to incompetence at the gastro-oesophageal barrier; (ii) damage to the oesophageal lining by irritant gastric contents; (iii) reduced oesophageal mucosal defence; (iv) impaired oesophageal motility with inadequate clearing of acidic refluxate above the gastro-oesophageal junction; and (v) delayed gastric emptying, which, in turn, causes an increase in gastric content volume and greater reflux [2–5]. In 50% of patients, the lower oesophageal sphincter pressure is recorded as normal during investigation and it is thought that the cause of reflux is transient reductions in pressure during varying times of the day.

Bile reflux is also thought to be a contributory factor. Aspirin, non-steroidal anti-inflammatory drugs (NSAIDs) and a number of foods (Table 2.1) can cause problems [6]. Recumbency, particularly during sleep, is a provocative factor. The role of a hiatus hernia remains uncertain but related problems may be due to a pooling of acid within the

Table 2.1 Food items associated with GORD [8].

Fatty foods
Chocolate
Carminatives (e.g. peppermint)
Alcohol
Citrus fruits
Tomato-based products
Coffee

hernia and delayed oesophageal emptying [7]. Hiatus hernia may also be linked with a further reduction of gastro-oesophageal incompetence and reduced lower oesophageal pressure. Psychological factors have been indirectly linked with GORD, particularly symptoms of globus, and non-cardiac pain. Although the mechanism of psychological effect upon gastro-oesophageal reflux is poorly understood, behavioural techniques have been used successfully to modify gastrointestinal function.

The relevance of *Helicobacter pylori* in GORD

There is no direct relationship between *Helicobacter pylori* and GORD. However, emerging work suggests that the eradication of *H. pylori* in dyspeptic patients may be associated with an increase in the prevalence of oesophagitis. The mechanisms remain unclear and controversial, and may be related to ascending changes in gastric mucosa or alterations in gastrin levels as a result of eradication.

Chest pain of oesophageal origin

The pathophysiology of non-cardiac chest pain remains unclear. Ten to thirty per cent of patients with suspected angina do not have demonstrable ischaemic heart disease, and as many as 60% of these are estimated to have pain of oesophageal origin, although not necessarily due to reflux.

The extent of the problem

Gastro-oesophageal reflux disease is a remarkably common problem. Community surveys have suggested a 10-year prevalence of 65% and a survey of symptoms within the previous 6 months indicated a prevalence of heartburn of 40% in the general population [9]. An American study has indicated that 7% of the population has daily heartburn and 36% suffer symptoms at least once a month. In addition, up to 50% of patients with non-cardiac chest pain, 60% of those with hoarseness and 80% of patients with chronic obstructive airways disease are affected by GORD [10]. It is likely that less than half of all sufferers seek medical advice.

In British general practice around 9% of all consultations are for gastrointestinal problems, half of which are related to the duodenum, stomach or oesophagus. Problems ascribed to the oesophagus (mainly oesophagitis) account for 103 per 10 000 consultations and are commonest in the 65–74 age group, and in females [11].

Presentation and common symptoms

Symptoms of GORD

The traditional symptoms of GORD are heartburn or regurgitation, especially after a large or fatty meal, aggravated by lying flat or bending. Associated symptoms include chronic hoarseness, asthma and chronic cough [12].

The natural history and progression of oesophagitis

Gastro-oesophageal reflux disease characteristically persists for years with episodes of spontaneous remission and relapses [13]. Oesophagitis waxes and wanes spontaneously. Some studies have shown a progression to a more severe grade of inflammation in a fifth of patients, whilst nearly half had no further episodes of oesophagitis after the initial episode [14]. Complications in patients referred to hospital with erosive oesophagitis are stricture in 4–20%, ulceration in 2–7%, haemorrhage in <2% and Barrett's oesophagus in 10–15%. In up to 10% of patients, oesophageal stricture is the presenting problem without a prior diagnosis of reflux oesophagitis.

Barrett's oesophagus and complications

Barrett's oesophagus is a complication of oesophagitis. It affects 10–15% of patients with oesophagitis and is thought to be the result of the repeated repair process at the site of inflammation. The hallmark of

Barrett's oesophagus is the formation of columnar epithelium and the condition has a high predisposition to adenocarcinoma. Neither symptom frequency nor severity is predictive of the extent of mucosal damage but there is a rising prevalence of Barrett's oesophagus with age. Although not all patients with Barrett's oesophagus will have had previously detected erosive oesophagitis, nearly all have a history of long-standing heartburn [14].

Clinical diagnosis and investigations

How accurate is a clinical diagnosis?

Although heartburn and regurgitation are indicators of GORD there is considerable overlap in symptoms from the upper, mid and lower gastrointestinal tract [15]. Symptoms relating to peptic ulcers, gallbladder disease and bowel problems lack sufficient specificity to allow a clinical diagnosis for GORD to be unequivocal on history alone, and GORD may coexist with other problems. None the less, the positive predictive value of a clinical diagnosis of GORD is higher than that of peptic ulcer disease or upper gastrointestinal cancer, and approaches 50% if endoscopic oesophagitis alone is seen as the confirmatory finding, compared with 22% for peptic ulcer and 4% for cancer [16]. In studies where heartburn or regurgitation is the predominant complaint, there is a high specificity for GORD defined as excessive acid exposure (89% and 95%, respectively, for heartburn and regurgitation), but a low sensitivity (38% and 6%, respectively) [17,18].

A further clinical diagnostic handicap is that, even when GORD is confirmed, expected symptoms such as heartburn may be absent. Up to 30% of patients with severe reflux with endoscopic findings may not suffer heartburn [19].

Is it safe to diagnose GORD on clinical grounds alone?

There is no unequivocal primary-care evidence establishing the security of a clinical diagnosis. A major problem is lack of agreement on the methodology of symptom scoring and endoscopic appearances. None the less, most specialists accept that a working diagnosis is likely to be reliable, particularly in young patients and in those who have no concurrent worrying symptoms. Such symptoms include vomiting, weight loss or bleeding. Gastro-oesophageal reflux disease may coexist with other lesions such as peptic ulcers or cholelithiasis, these being commoner in patients beyond their fourth decade, even if the predominant symptoms are positional heartburn and regurgitation.

Investigations: how appropriate and useful?

1 Gastroscopy

Gastroscopy remains valuable for detecting oesophagitis, defined as morphological change in the oesophagus ascribed to acid exposure. However, it may miss up to 50% of patients with reflux disease who do not have the morphological changes of oesophagitis. Whilst damage to the oesophageal mucosa, indicated by erosions or ulceration, correlates well with histological findings, non-specific appearances of redness and oedema are less reliable indicators of GORD [18]. The reporting of a raised gastro-oesophageal junction may be an indication of a hiatus hernia but cannot be interpreted as a sign of GORD. A function of endoscopy is to exclude concurrent lesions in patients with a clinical diagnosis of GORD.

Barium meal examinations are less frequently used for diagnosing GORD, partly because they may miss mild oesophagitis and also because the demonstration of reflux from abdominal pressure by the operator may be an inconsistent finding. It is indicated in patients with dysphagia.

2 Ambulatory pH monitoring

This measures the level of acidity in the oesophagus as an indicator of reflux. The percentage of time during which the pH is less than 4 and the day/night timing of episodes is used as a measure of GORD. This investigation is especially useful when the diagnosis remains doubtful after a normal endoscopy, and a correlation between symptoms and episodes of reduced pH is a confirmatory factor for GORD.

3 Oesophageal manometry

This is used to assess oesophageal peristaltic action, particularly if specific oesophageal motor disorders such as achalasia or neuromuscular dysfunction related to multiple sclerosis are suspected.

4 *The diagnostic acid suppression test*

This reflects everyday general practice. The use of high-dose acid suppression therapy with proton pump inhibitors (PPIs) in patients in whom the predominant symptom is heartburn without complications has been mooted as a diagnostic test. Resolution of symptoms points to the problem being GORD. High-dose acid suppression with a PPI virtually eliminates gastric acid production and, in theory, abolishes reflux symptoms [20]. However, as the specificity of heartburn as a symptom of GORD is not 100%, there is the risk of overlap with other acid-sensitive disorders.

Management

(i) Lifestyle measures

Overweight patients may benefit from weight reduction and a reduction in fat intake relieves symptoms [21]. Elevation of the head of the bed by 6 inches, although not always practical, has been reported to improve symptoms and heal oesophagitis [22]. Smoking, coffee, alcohol and chocolate are known to provoke reflux and fruit juices and spicy foods can irritate inflamed mucosa.

(ii) Antacids and alginates

Antacids work by raising the pH of stomach contents and alginates by forming a floating layer as a physical barrier to reflux. Placebo-controlled trials of antacid in the treatment of reflux have shown no or slight benefit only and no improvements in endoscopic appearances [23]. In one 3-year study the prolonged use of regular antacids combined with lifestyle measures did not lead to the healing of oesophagitis, but symptom relief has been noted in around 20% of patients over a prolonged period [24,25].

Alginates have been shown to relieve symptoms more effectively than antacids [23] in controlled trials, but no studies have shown healing of oesophagitis with alginate alone. In one large study of patients with oesophagitis who had initial healing therapy, 76% remained relapse free for 6 months when maintained with alginates.

(iii) Mucosal protection therapy

Sucralfate is a topically active aluminium hydroxide salt. It forms a physical barrier by adhering to damaged tissue. Symptom relief and healing rates are comparable to that with H_2-receptor antagonists (H_2RAs) in comparative trials, but, paradoxically the superiority of sucralfate over placebo has been demonstrated only in a minority of trials [26]. Sucralfate does not appear successful in relapse prevention or in maintenance treatment.

(iv) Motility-altering drugs

Prokinetic drugs such as metoclopramide and domperidone work by stimulating the upper gastrointestinal tract, and cisapride by stimulating the entire gastrointestinal tract. Metoclopromide is a dopamine antagonist which increases lower oesophageal pressure, decreases gastro-oesophageal reflux and accelerates gastric emptying. At a dose of 10 mg before meals it has been demonstrated to be superior to placebo and as effective as H_2RAs in conventional doses [27]. Healing of oesophagitis has not been convincingly shown by metoclopramide alone but healing rates are accelerated when H_2RAs are used concurrently [28]. Dose-related side effects, mainly lethargy as well as extraprydimal symptoms, limit the use of metoclopramide. Domperidone has a similar action to metoclopramide but fewer side effects. Inconsistent results have been obtained from its use in GORD.

Cisapride is commonly used in many European countries and the USA for the management of GORD. It functions by increasing lower oesophageal pressure, stimulating contractions in the oesophagus and stomach, and it also improves antro-duodenal co-ordination to improve clearance through the pylorus. It acts throughout the gut as opposed to the upper gut for metoclopramide and domperidone. Cisapride has been shown to be effective in reducing symptoms of reflux and promotes healing in patients with GORD and oesophagitis [26]. Cisapride at 20/40 mg daily has been found to be comparable to ranitidine 300 mg daily in symptom relief and healing rates, and the effects of H_2RAs have been shown, in controlled studies, to be enhanced by the addition of cisapride [26]. Relapse rates after initial healing therapy are also reduced by using cisapride [26]. However, cardiac side effects limit their use in some patients.

(v) Acid suppression drugs

H_2-receptor blockers and proton pump inhibitors

H_2-receptor antagonists work by decreasing acid output. Numerous studies have confirmed the safety and efficacy of H_2RAs in reducing the symptoms of GORD, but some 35–40% of patients do not experience symptom relief [29,30]. Between 40 and 60% of patients with reflux oesophagitis do not experience full mucosal healing at standard doses [31], and even symptom relief requires greater acid suppression than is needed for patients with peptic ulcer. To achieve healing of oesophagitis, higher doses than for symptom relief may be needed [32]. Most studies have utilized standard doses of H_2RAs (cimetidine 400 mg q.d.s.; ranitidine or nizatidine 150 mg b.d.). At these doses heartburn is relieved in 50% of patients at 4 weeks and oesophagitis healing occurs in 30% at 4 weeks, with the best results in patients with mild symptoms or findings. Higher doses, e.g. ranitidine 150 mg q.d.s., heal mild oesophagitis in 80% of patients at 8 weeks and severe oesophagitis in 70% at 12 weeks [32]. The concurrent use of prokinetic drugs (see above) reduces gastro-oesophageal reflux and has a synergistic action to the H_2RAs.

Proton pump inhibitors produce a greater degree of acid suppression than H_2RAs and are commonly used in GORD in treating acute episodes and for long-term management. Their efficacy is a class effect with few major differences between different products, although most available research relates to omeprazole and lansoprazole. Omeprazole at 20 mg has been shown to produce rapid relief of heartburn and healing in oesophagitis in 65% of patients at 4 weeks, and up to 85% at 8 weeks [33]. Omeprazole at 40 mg daily is more effective in those who have not responded to 20 mg [34,35]. Lansoprazole has been demonstrated as healing oesophagitis in 89% of patients at 8 weeks [36].

The superiority of PPIs over H_2RAs has been clearly established for both symptom relief and healing of oesophagitis, in the short and the long term [33]. This applies particularly to patients who have not responded to H_2RAs at standard doses. In one study, PPIs relieved symptoms and produced healing in 86% and 90%, respectively, at 8 weeks, compared with 32% and 47% with H_2RAs. An analysis of over 30 randomized controlled trials [12] confirms this superiority in all grades of symptoms, and a recent UK-based Bandolier report established the 'numbers needed to treat' (NNT) ratio for omeprazole vs. ranitidine at over 3 for short-term healing and 2.8 for long-term maintenance.

There is a paucity of general-practice-based data on the effect of lower doses of PPIs for symptom control and oesophagitis healing, but many patients are adequately controlled on omeprazole 10 mg or lansoprazole 15 mg. At the same time it is known that a proportion of patients continue to secrete acid despite high doses of PPI (e.g. omeprazole 40 mg b.d.) and do not experience symptom relief and healing.

Potential problems with using PPIs

The profound level of acid suppression produced by PPIs initially led some to fear long-term consequences, e.g. from the overgrowth of bacteria in the stomach. Evidence to date confirms the safety of PPI therapy even in long-term usage. There have been suggestions that increase in gastrin levels may occur as a result of PPI therapy, although the clinical effect of this is unclear. Where patients have been treated for 8–12 weeks with omeprazole, the recurrence of symptoms and oesophagitis has been reported in up to 60% of patients at 4 months and in 82% at 6 months [37], suggesting that one consequence of PPI therapy may be an increase in acid-producing cells and rebound acid hypersecretion.

(vi) Surgical management

Laparscopic surgical management offers a real alternative to drug therapy, particularly in patients with severe or poorly responsive symptoms. The commonest procedure is Nissen fundoplication or a variation, in which the distal oesophagus is anchored below the diaphragm by wrapping the gastric fundus around the distal oesophagus. This also has the effect of constructing a valve mechanism to prevent reflux. In expert hands an efficacy of 90% has been reported [38]. Complications include splenic trauma leading to open splenectomy, vagal damage, dysphagia, and the 'gas bloat syndrome' in which the patient has difficulty belching or vomiting as a consequence of a tight sphincter.

Results of comparison between antireflux surgery and medical treatment are difficult to compare. A controlled trial comparing surgery with ranitidine, metoclopramide and sucralfate showed that patients with oesophagitis, stricture or Barrett's metaplasia did better with surgery at the end of 1 year [38]. However, comparisons of PPIs with surgery are awaited.

2

Management of Barrett's oesophagus

Barrett's oesophagus, leading to metaplastic changes, is the result of chronic gastro-oesophageal reflux (see p. 11). The prevalence of Barrett's oesophagus is rising, and although it is essentially managed in secondary care there are implications for general practitioners with regard to its detection and follow-up. The link between Barrett's metaplasia and adenocarcinoma sets it as a premalignant condition, with the relative risk of carcinoma estimated at 30- to 40-fold [38]. Management is centred on treating the reflux and planned surveillance of patients with established Barrett's oesophagus. The incidence of adenocarcinoma in Western countries is increasing, currently at 3/100 000, although not all of this is linked to Barrett's oesophagus.

The management of Barrett's oesophagus is based on antireflux measures with PPIs or surgery. Regression of Barrett's metaplasia can occur even though the metaplastic tissue may persist. High-dose acid suppression therapy with laser or photodynamic ablation of the metaplastic tissue has been tried, but the effectiveness has not been ascertained. Controversy also exists as to how often patients with Barrett's oesophagus should undergo repeated endoscopies and biopsies, and recommendations range from 6 months to 2-yearly intervals dependent upon initial findings and progress [38].

Long-term therapy in GORD

There is less certainty about the long-term management of GORD than about acute management. Many authorities accept that, if an endoscopic diagnosis of GORD has been established, follow-up endoscopies are not required unless problems develop or Barrett's oesophagus was discovered. Treatment can be geared to symptom relief. As it is likely that as many as 90% of patients will relapse within 6 months of a healing course of therapy [39], the question also arises as to whether treatment can be used intermittently rather than continuously. Evidence suggests that more than 50% of patients on long-term repeat prescriptions for PPIs only take their medication intermittently [40,41]. Formal studies investigating the possibility of PPIs taken on alternative days or weekends alone have not demonstrated efficacy [42].

Long-term management of GORD with H_2RAs has been disappointing compared with cisapride or PPIs. Low-dose H_2RAs (e.g. 150 mg ranitidine) are comparable only to placebo. Ten milligrams of omeprazole has been shown to be superior to placebo but less effective

Table 2.2 Treatment options.

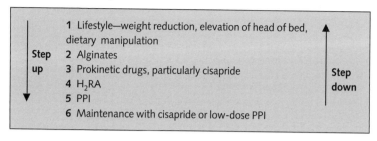

Step up	1 Lifestyle—weight reduction, elevation of head of bed, dietary manipulation 2 Alginates 3 Prokinetic drugs, particularly cisapride 4 H₂RA 5 PPI 6 Maintenance with cisapride or low-dose PPI	Step down

than 20 mg daily [42]. Low-dose cisapride (10 mg b.d.) has been shown to be effective in long-term management. Lansoprazole has been shown to be effective at 30 mg and at 15 mg in a proportion of patients requiring maintenance.

'Step-up' or 'step-down' therapy?

The principle of 'step-up' therapy is to commence the patient on the least powerful and, by implication, the least expensive therapy and to step up as required in response to symptoms and findings. In contrast 'step-down' therapy entails initial management with the most efficacious drug and a stepwise reduction to a level that contains symptoms with less powerful and cheaper drugs (Table 2.2). In addition to rationalization by therapeutic classes of drugs, these approaches acknowledge the cost element of treating GORD in an increasingly cost-limited health system. Although drug costs alone are easily computable, the overall comparisons of these two approaches are made more complex if quality of life, symptom control assessments, health-related economic losses and consultation costs are included.

The advantage of the step-up regimen is possible avoidance of expensive drugs, particularly in long-term use, whilst the chief disadvantage is delay in instituting an appropriate level of therapy. A step-down approach allows a faster control of symptoms and healing, but has the inherent disadvantage that many patients will find it difficult to relinquish the more powerful drugs. There is an absence of primary-care trials comparing the two approaches.

References

1 de Boer WA, Tytgat GNJ. Review article: drug therapy for reflux oesophagitis. *Aliment Pharmacol Ther* 1994; **8** (2): 147–57.

2 Castell DO. Esophagitis: a motility disorder? *Motility* 1989; **2**: 4.
3 Radmark T, Petterson GB. Lower oesophageal sphincter pressure in normal individuals and patients with gastro-oesophageal reflux. *Scand J Gastroenterol* 1989; **24**: 842–50.
4 Price SF, Smithson KW, Castell DO. Food sensitivity on reflux oesophagitis. *Gastroenterology* 1978; **75**: 240–3.
5 Lloyd DA, Borda IT. Food-induced heartburn: the effect of osmolality. *Gastroenterology* 1981; **80**: 740–1.
6 Little AG, DeMeester TR, Kirchner PT, O'Sullivan GC, Skinner DB. Pathogenesis of oesophagitis in patients with gastro-oespphageal reflux. *Surgery* 1980; **88**: 101–7.
7 Sloan S, Rademaker RW, Kahrilas PJ. Determinants of gastro-oesophageal incompetence: hiatal hernia, lower oesophageal sphincter, or both? *Ann Intern Med* 1992; **117**: 977–82.
8 Fisher RS. Gastro-oesophageal reflux disease: acute and chronic treatment. In: Champion MC, Orr WC, eds. *Gastrointestinal Motility*. Oxford: Blackwell Science, 1996.
9 Jones RH, Lydeard SE, Hobbs FDR. Dyspepsia in England and Scotland. *Gut* 1990; **31**: 401–5.
10 Sontag SJ, O'Connell S, Khandelval S, Miller T. Most asthmatics have gastro-oesophageal reflux with or without bronchodilator therapy. *Gastroenterology* 1990; **99**(3): 613–20.
11 *Morbidity Statistics from General Practice*. HMSO, 1995.
12 DeVault KR, Castell D. Guidelines for the diagnosis and treatment of gastro-oesophageal reflux disease. *Arch Intern Med* 1995; **155**: 2165–73.
13 Schindlbeck NE, Klauser AG, Berghammer G. Three-year follow-up of patients with gastro-oesophageal reflux disease. *Gut* 1992; **33**: 1016–19.
14 Ollyo JB, Monnier Fontolliet C. The natural history, prevalence and incidence of reflux oesophagitis. *Gullet* 1993; **3** (suppl.): 3–10.
15 Armstrong D, Bennet JR, Blum AL. The endoscopic assessment of oesophagitis: a progress report on observer agreement. *Gastroenterology* 1996; **111**: 85–92.
16 Hungin APS, Bramble MG, Idle N. Is it possible to diagnose dyspepsia accurately in general practice? *Gut* 1997; **40** (S1): F28.
17 Klauser AG, Schindlebeck NE, Muller-Lissner SA. Symptoms in gastro-oesophageal reflux disease. *Lancet* 1990; **335**: 205–8.
18 Johnsson F, Joelsson B, Dodmundsson K. Symptoms and endoscopic findings in the diagnosis of gastro-oesophageal reflux disease. *Scand J Gastroenterol* 1987; **22**: 714–18.
19 Johnson DA, Winters C, Spurling TJ. Esophageal acid sensitivity in Barrett's oesophagus. *J Clin Gastroenterol* 1987; **9**: 23–7.
20 Klauser AG, Voderholzer WA, Muller-Lissner SA. Is empiric acid suppression of diagnostic value in gastro-oesophageal reflux disease? *Gastroenterology* 1993; **104**: A22.
21 Kuster E, Ros E, Toledo-Pimentel V. Predictive factors of the long term outcome in gastro-oesophageal reflux disease: six year follow-up of 107 patients. *Gut* 1994; **35**: 8–14.
22 Harvey RF, Hadley N, Gill TR. Effects of sleeping with the bed head raised and of ranitidine in patients with severe peptic oesophagitis. *Lancet* 1987; **ii**: 1200–3.

23 Scarpignato C, Galmiche J-P. Antacids and alginates. In: Rozen P, Scarpignato C, eds. *The Treatment of Gastro-Oesophagael Reflux Disease*. Basel: Karger, 1992, pp. 153–81.

24 Behar J, Sheahan DG, Biancani P. Medical and surgical treatment of reflux oesophagitis. A 38 month report on a prospective clinical trial. *N Eng J Med* 1975; **293**: 263–8.

25 Lieberman DA. Medical therapy for chronic reflux oesophagitis: long term follow up. *Arch Intern Med* 1987; **147**: 717–20.

26 Tytgat G, Janssens Reynolds JC. Update on the pathophysiology and management of gastro-oesophageal reflux disease: the role of prokinetic therapy. *Eur J Gastroenterol Hepatol* 1996; **8**: 603–11.

27 Scarpignato C, Guslandi M. Metoclopramide: is there still a place in the treatment of gastro-oesophageal reflux disease? In: Rozen P, Scarpignato C, eds., *The Treatment of Gastro-Oesophageal Reflux Disease*. Basel: Karger 1992: 17–29.

28 Wiseman LR, Faulds D. Cisapride: An updated review of its pharmacology and therapeutic efficacy as a prokinetic agent in gastrointestinal motility disorders. *Drugs* 1994; **47**: 116–52.

29 Colin-Jones DJ. H_2 receptor antagonists in gastro-oesophageal reflux. *Gut* 1989; **30**: 1305–8.

30 Pope CE II. Acid-reflux disorders. *N Engl J Med* 1914; **331**: 656–60.

31 Klinkenberg-Knol EC, Jansen JMBJ, Festen HPM. Double blind multi-centre comparison of omeprazole and ranitidine in the treatment of reflux oesophagitis. *Lancet* 1987; **i**: 349–51.

32 Roufail W, Belsito A, Robinson M. Ranitidine for erosive oesophagitis: a double-blind placebo controlled study. *Aliment Pharmacol Ther* 1992; **6**: 597–607.

33 Bandolier. Oxford, February 1997; **36**: 3.

34 Sandmark S, Carlson R, Fausa O. Omeprazole or ranitidine in the treatment of reflux oesophagitis. *Scand J Gastroenterol* 1988; **23**: 625–32.

35 Dent Y, Yeomans ND, Mackinnon M. Omeprazole v ranitidine for prevention of relapse in reflux oesophagitis. *Gut* 1994; **35**: 590–8.

36 Sontag SJ. Gastro-oesophageal reflux disease. *Aliment Pharmacol Ther* 1993; **7**: 293–312.

37 Ang ST, Leiberman DA, Ippolti AF. Long-term omeprazole therapy in patients with Barrett's oesophagus is associated with parietal cell hyperplasia. *Gastroenterology* 1994; **106**: A1016.

38 Kahrilas PJ. Gastro-oesophageal reflux disease. *JAMA* 1996; **276**: 983–92.

39 Hetzel DJ, Dent J, Reed WD. Healing and relapse of severe peptic oesophagitis after treatment with omeprazole. *Gastroenterology* 1988; **95**: 903–12.

40 Hungin AP, Rubin GP, O'Flanagan H. Long-term prescribing of PPIs in general practice. *Br J Gen Pract* 1999; **49**: 451–3.

41 Hungin AP, Rubin GP, O'Flanagan H. Factors influencing compliance in long-term PPI therapy in general practice. *Br J Gen Pract* 1999; **49**: 463–4.

42 Bank S, Magier D, Greenberg R. Alternate day omeprazole maintenance therapy in H_2RA resistant oesophagitis. *Gastroenterology* 1992; **102**: A35.

2

3 Dyspepsia and *Helicobacter pylori*

Greg Rubin

Key Points

- 40% of the general population experience dyspepsia in a 12-month period; less than 10% have peptic ulcer disease.
- Symptoms are a poor predictor of peptic ulcer disease.
- Investigate patients with alarm symptoms or new symptoms at age over 45, or those who relapse after treatment.
- Treatment is by *Helicobacter pylori* eradication when appropriate, or with acid-suppressing drugs.

Background

Peptic ulcer disease (PUD) is a major cause of ill health in developed countries. It affects about 10% of adult males, and fewer females, at some time in their lives, and is responsible for 4500 deaths per annum in the UK. The point prevalence of active PUD is 1–2%, although even in an apparently normal healthy population the point prevalence is 1%. The incidence of duodenal ulcer is about 0.18% per year, and increases with age to 0.3% for men in their 70s. Gastric ulcer is less common, with an incidence of 0.03%.

Incidence rates have declined markedly in the past three decades, though hospitalization rates for complications of PUD have not shown significant change. Furthermore, perforation and death rates have increased among women aged 60 or over, in parallel with an increase in the use of non-steroidal anti-inflammatory drugs (NSAIDs) in this age group [1].

Non-ulcer dyspepsia (NUD) is a very much more common disorder. A large community survey in southern England found a 6-month incidence for dyspepsia of 38%, of whom a quarter consulted their doctor.

Table 3.1 What causes dyspepsia?

Helicobacter pylori
Acid and pepsin secretion
Alcohol
Drugs
Cigarette smoking
Genetic factors
Psychological factors

The incidence of dyspepsia in the community is 10–11% per annum, but the rate of PUD is 0.5%. In other words, over 90% of all incident cases of dyspepsia are suffering from NUD or gastro-oesophageal reflux disease.

The evidence to link diet to the development of peptic ulcer is fragmentary, although coffee and cola drinks consumption are associated with increased prevalence of duodenal ulcer. There is a well-proven independent association between smoking and ulcer disease [2]. No general conclusion can be reached on the significance of acid and pepsin secretion in the pathogenesis of petic ulcer. An imbalance between these factors, together with changes in mucosal resistance, is likely to be important for at least some patients.

Aspirin and NSAIDs are well known as causes of both acute gastric mucosal damage and chronic ulceration. Endoscopic studies have repeatedly shown an excess of both duodenal and gastric ulcers in patients taking NSAIDs, and their use is associated with haemorrhage and perforation. The risk of these complications increases two- to four-fold in the elderly, and is more marked in women.

Although there is no direct evidence that *Helicobacter pylori* infection precedes the development of duodenal ulcer, it produces an exaggerated gastrin response, duodenitis and gastritis. Over 90% of patients with duodenal ulcer not associated with NSAID use have *H. pylori* infection, as do over 70% of those with gastric ulcer [3]. The population-attributable risk for *H. pylori* is 48% and *H. pylori* is the most important individual risk factor for peptic ulcer. The association between *H. pylori* and NUD, however, is unclear and is based on a limited benefit observed in some, but not all, trials of eradication therapy.

It is not possible to draw clear distinctions between most of the causative factors for PUD and NUD.

Table 3.2 Indications for early investigation.

New dyspepsia at age >45
Recurrent symptoms after adequate therapy
Recurrent symptoms from a known gastric ulcer
Presence of alarm symptoms:
    dysphagia
    vomiting
    weight loss
    bleeding
    anaemia

3

Presentation and investigation

Dyspepsia has been defined as upper abdominal or retrosternal pain or discomfort referable to the upper gastrointestinal tract. Attempts have been made to define sub-sets of dyspeptic symptoms that correlate to specific diagnoses. Unfortunately these are little better than chance in predicting PUD. Symptom interpretation is made difficult by the intermittent nature of the condition, the lack of correlation between symptom severity and the decision to seek medical help, and the existence of peptic ulcers in patients who are apparently symptom free. The decision to investigate a patient with dyspepsia is one determined by the patient's beliefs and concerns as well as the clinical history.

Some features should prompt you to consider investigation at an early stage [4] (Table 3.2).

Patients with alarm symptoms require prompt endoscopic investigation to establish a diagnosis. The relative risk of serious disease (ulcers or cancer) is greater in patients presenting with one or more alarm symptoms compared with patients without such symptoms, although the absolute risks remain low in a primary health-care population [5].

Older patients should be sent for endoscopy because the relative risk of gastro-oesophageal malignancy increases with age. The age cut-off is arbitrarily defined and varies between countries. Age >45 years is recommended, although it is recognized that even then the absolute risk of malignancies in dyspeptic patients will be low. Fewer than 5% of gastric cancers occur in patients aged under 45 years [6]. Indeed, for patients with uncomplicated dyspepsia 55 years has been shown to be a safe cut-off point [7].

3

The timing of investigation in those patients whose symptoms do not give rise to immediate concern is an important health resource issue. Several studies of alternative management strategies for dyspepsia have demonstrated that early endoscopy is the most cost-effective approach. Even when endoscopy is initially deferred, 70% of patients will end up being investigated within 1 year [8].

More recently, tests for *H. pylori* have been used as a first step in the investigation of patients with dyspepsia. When used to select patients for gastroscopy, the 'test and endoscope strategy', this is effective in reducing the rate of investigation by around 20%. Much more common is the use of these tests to select patients for eradication therapy—the 'test and treat' strategy.

The evidence to support a 'test and treat' strategy remains inconclusive. Issues that may influence its effectiveness include the prevalence of *H. pylori* infection and of PUD, the predictive value of *H. pylori* tests and the clinical effectiveness of the strategy.

When should *H. pylori* eradication be considered?

The primary care scenarios in which *H. pylori* eradication should be considered are shown in Table 3.3. It is advisable not to test for *H. pylori* unless you intend to treat or refer for endoscopy should the result be positive.

Patients with a new diagnosis of duodenal ulcer, and those with a previously diagnosed duodenal ulcer who become symptomatic or are taking long-term antisecretory therapy, should receive eradication therapy without *H. pylori* testing. Patients with a new diagnosis of gastric ulcer, and those with a previously diagnosed gastric ulcer who become symptomatic or are taking long-term antisecretory therapy, should be tested for *H. pylori* infection and given eradication therapy if appropriate.

H. pylori eradication reduces ulcer recurrence rates at 1 year to 6% (vs. 67% for patients not cured of *H. pylori* infection) and 4% for gastric ulcer (vs. 59% for patients not cured of *H. pylori* infection) [10]. *H. pylori* eradication in patients with duodenal ulcer produces more rapid healing [11] and a higher rate of healing.

Although consensus statements have recommended eradication as first-line therapy in *H. pylori*-associated peptic ulceration on clinical [5] and cost-effectiveness grounds [12], delay of therapy until the first ulcer relapse has also been advocated. This is based on the fact that 20–40% of ulcers in patients with *H. pylori* do not recur, possibly because of the existence of other risk factors such as smoking [13].

Table 3.3 When and how to test for *H. pylori* infection [9].

Patient presentation	Test for H. pylori?
Patients with alarm symptoms (weight loss, vomiting, haematemesis, anaemia, dysphagia) or aged >45 with new dyspepsia	No, prompt endoscopy advised
Uninvestigated dyspepsia	
First presentation	Routine testing for *H. pylori* not recommended
Subsequent presentations due to symptom relapse	'Test and treat' or 'Test and endoscope'
Patients with a previous endoscopic diagnosis	
Non-ulcer dyspepsia	Routine testing not recommended
Duodenal ulcer	
New diagnosis	Prescribe *H. pylori* eradication
Previous diagnosis and now symptomatic	therapy without prior testing
Currently taking long-term acid-suppression therapy	
After *H. pylori* eradication therapy	Testing not routinely necessary
Gastric ulcer	
New diagnosis	Test to confirm *H. pylori*
Previous diagnosis and now symptomatic	infection before treating
Currently taking long-term acid-suppression therapy	
After *H. pylori* eradication therapy	Confirm cure and eradication by endoscopy
Other situations	
Recurrent dyspepsia after *H. pylori* eradication therapy	Test with urea breath test
Relatives of *H. pylori*-infected patients	Not recommended

3

H. pylori testing and eradication are not recommended for patients with NUD. Individual studies of the benefit of *H. pylori* eradication in patients with NUD are mostly flawed, with sub-optimal study design, unclear presentation of data, heterogeneity of results and lack of consensus on outcome measures. In particular there is no standardized method of measuring symptom improvement [14]. Much of the literature is inappropriate to primary care as most research takes place in highly selected hospital populations, or is of cohort study quality [13]. As a result, systematic reviews of the literature largely conclude that no firm conclusions can be drawn on the benefits of *H. pylori* eradication in *H. pylori*-positive patients with NUD [15,16]. More recent studies have failed to resolve the uncertainty that exists [17,18].

There is evidence for clustering of *H. pylori* infection in families [19]. However, many infected individuals do not have dyspepsia and on this basis testing and treatment of family members are not advocated.

Testing for *Helicobacter pylori*

The use and choice of test for *H. pylori* need careful consideration (Table 3.4). The ^{13}C-urea breath test (CUBT), histology and the rapid urease (CLO) test are the gold standard diagnostic tests for *H. pylori* infection. These all identify active infection and may be used for initial diagnosis. The CUBT may give false-negative results in the presence of proton pump inhibitor (PPI) drugs, antibiotics or bismuth [20]. Serological tests demonstrate seroconversion 22–33 days after infection. They also require local validation against sera from patients with a predeter-mined *H. pylori* status. A meta-analysis of 21 studies of serological kits for *H. pylori* infection found that overall, at a sensitivity of 85%, specificity was estimated to be 79%. It concluded that the overall accuracy of these kits may not be adequate for decision making in all patient groups [21].

Routine confirmation of eradication is not required, but should be undertaken in those who presented with a history of complicated ulcer (bleeding or perforation). Patients with gastric ulcer should have a repeat endoscopy when ulcer healing can be confirmed and a CLO test performed. Patients who present with recurrent dyspepsia after a course of *H. pylori* eradication therapy should be tested by CUBT to determine whether further eradication treatment is indicated. Re-infection is uncommon in adults and recurrent symptoms are rarely due to this.

The CUBT, histology and CLO test are all also suitable for diagnosing successful eradication, which should be delayed for at least 4 weeks

Table 3.4 Tests fo *H. pylori* infection.

Office tests	Utility
^{13}C- or ^{14}C-urea breath test	For diagnosis: highly reliable NB Stop antisecretories, bismuth and antibiotics 2 weeks prior to test To confirm cure: highly reliable NB Test 4 weeks after end of treatment
Serology or whole blood, near patient test	For diagnosis: satisfactory To confirm cure: not suitable NB Be aware of the sensitivity and specificity of these tests
Hospital-based tests Laboratory based (ELISA)	For diagnosis: highly reliable but requires local validation To confirm cure: not suitable
^{13}C- or ^{14}C-urea breath test	See above
Endoscopy with biopsy for rapid urease test	For diagnosis: highly reliable To confirm cure: highly reliable

after the end of treatment [13]. Serological titres do not drop significantly until the sixth month after *H. pylori* has been eradicated. The need for paired sera also makes these tests less suitable for the demonstration of successful cure.

Treatment of dyspepsia

H. pylori *eradication therapy*

The published meta-analyses of eradication therapy trials reflect the rapid pace of change in this area of management. Early studies found bismuth-based triple therapies to be the most effective, but identified antibiotic resistance, side effects and drug compliance as important factors affecting efficacy [22]. More recently, a pooled, intention-to-treat analysis of 307 studies of eradication therapies concluded that PPI-based triple therapies were necessary to achieve eradication rates >80%, and that omeprazole/clarithromycin-based regimens were the

Table 3.5 Recommended treatments.

First-line H. pylori *eradication regimen* The recommended first-line eradication therapy is: PPI (standard dose) + clarithromycin (500 mg) + amoxycillin (1 g) All given twice daily for 1 week This will optimize the chances of eradication of *H. pylori* and minimize the risks of promoting metronidazole resistance *Alternative* H. pylori *eradication regimen* Where the prevalence of metronidazole resistance is low: PPI (standard dose) + clarithromycin (500 mg) + metronidazole (400 mg) All given twice daily for 1 week

most effective with a 87% success rate [23]. Key factors were identified as a short treatment course and twice daily dosing, although the ideal therapy still remained to be determined.

A more complex meta-analysis from North America included decision analytical modelling to determine costs and health outcomes [24]. This concluded that standard triple therapy plus proton pump inhibitor, and clarithromycin, metronidazole and PPI regimens had the highest compliance-adjusted eradication rates at 86% and 85% respectively (Table 3.5).

It should be remembered that the studies on which these meta-analyses are based have very largely been conducted in tightly defined settings and on populations drawn from secondary care. There are no meta-analyses of eradication studies conducted in primary care.

Studies of eradication therapy in NUD continue to produce conflicting results [17,18]. Overall, the response rate is around 30%, with some showing a benefit over placebo of up to 10%. At present, eradication therapy cannot be recommended for patients with NUD.

Antacids

Antacids neutralize gastric acid and raise the pH in the stomach. Alginate or raft antacids are designed for gastro-oesophageal reflux, have little neutralizing capacity and are ineffective in PUD.

Neutralizing antacids are cheap and have been a traditional first-line therapy for dyspepsia. They are effective healing agents particularly for duodenal ulcer, and have been shown to reduce relapse rate when taken as a maintenance therapy. The unwanted side effects, diarrhoea or constipation, electrolyte disturbances and drug interactions, together with their inconvenience, limit their usefulness.

Acid suppressing drugs

The advent of H_2-receptor antagonist drugs revolutionized the management of peptic ulcer. They remain widely used as maintenance therapy, despite increasing awareness of the importance of *H. pylori* eradication. Duodenal ulcer healing rates of 70–80% at 4 weeks and 90–95% at 8 weeks can be expected. Spontaneous relapse within 1 year can be reduced from 80% to 20% by continuing these drugs at half the healing doses.

H_2-receptor antagonists (H_2RAs) are widely used, often on an as needed basis, for functional dyspepsia. The therapeutic benefit can be difficult to predict although patients with ulcer-like dyspepsia might be expected to respond best to these drugs.

Proton pump inhibitor drugs inhibit the means by which acid is secreted and are potent acid suppressing agents. They achieve ulcer healing rates of over 90% at 4 weeks and also relieve symptoms more quickly than H_2RAs [25].

References

1 Bardhan KD, Cust G, Hinchcliffe RFC, Williamson FM, Lyon C, Bose K. Changing patterns of admissions and operations for duodenal ulcer. *Br J Surg* 1989; **79**: 230–6.
2 Friedman GD, Siegelaub AB, Seltzer CC. Cigarettes, alcohol, coffee and peptic ulcer. *N Engl J Med* 1974; **290**: 469–73.
3 Veldhuyzen van Zanten SJO, Sherman PM. *Helicobacter pylori* infection as a cause of gastritis, duodenal ulcer, gastric cancer and non-ulcer dyspepsia; a systematic overview. *Can Med Assoc J* 1994; **150** (2): 177–85.
4 British Society of Gastroenterology. *Provision of Gastrointestinal Endoscopy and Related Services for a District General Hospital.* London: British Society of Gastroenterology, 1990.
5 Meineche-Schmidt V, Jorgensen T. Prognosis of dyspepsia among patients in general practice. The consequence of having one or more alarm symptoms. *Gastroenterology* 1996; **110**: A29.
6 Association of Comprehensive Cancer Centres. *Incidence of Cancer in the Netherlands.* Utrecht 1998.
7 Christie J, Shepherd NA, Codling BW, Valori RM. Gastric cancer below the age of 55: implications for screening patients with uncomplicated dyspepsia. *Gut* 1997; **41**: 513–17.

8 Bytzer P, Hansen JM, de Muckadell OBS. Empirical H$_2$ blocker therapy or prompt endoscopy in management of dyspepsia. *Lancet* 1994; **343**: 811–16.

9 Rubin GP, Meineche-Schmidt V, Roberts AP, Childe SM, de Wit NJ. The management of *Helicobacter pylori* infection in primary care. Guidelines from the European Society for Primary Care Gastroenterology. *Eur J Gen Pract* 1999; **5**: 98–104.

10 Hopkins RJ, Girardi LS, Turney E. Relationship between *Helicobacter pylori* eradication and reduced duodenal and gastric ulcer recurrence: a review. *Gastroenterology* 1996; **110**: 1244–52.

11 Veldhuyzen van Zanten SJ, Sherman PM. Indications for treatment of *H. pylori*: a systematic overview. *Can Med Assoc J* 1994; **150** (2): 189–98.

12 O'Brien B, Goeree R, Mohamed H, Hunt R. Cost-effectiveness of *Helicobacter pylori* eradication for the long-term management of duodenal ulcer in Canada. *Arch Intern Med* 1995; **155**: 1958–64.

13 Delaney BC. Role of *H. pylori* in gastrointestinal disease: implications for primary care of a revolution in the management of dyspepsia. *Br J Gen Pract* 1995; **45**: 489–94.

14 Veldhuyzen van Zanten SJ, Cleary C, Talley NJ *et al.* Drug treatment of functional dyspepsia: a systematic analysis of trial methodology with recommendations of designs for future trials. *Am J Gastroenterol* 1996; **91** (4): 660–73.

15 Lahej RJ, Jansen B, van de Lisdonk EH, Severens JL, Verbeek AL. Symptom improvement through eradication of *H. pylori* in patients with non-ulcer dyspepsia. *Aliment Pharmacol Ther* 1996; **10**: 843–50.

16 Talley NJA. Critique of therapeutic trials in *H. pylori* positive functional dyspepsia. *Gastroenterology* 1994; **106** (5): 1174–83.

17 McColl K, Murray L, El-Omar E *et al.* Symptomatic benefit from eradicating *Helicobacter pylori* infection in patients with non-ulcer dyspepsia. *N Engl J Med* 1998; **26**: 1869–74.

18 Blum A, Talley NJ, O'Morain C *et al.* Lack of effect of treating *Helicobacter pylori* infection in patients with non-ulcer dyspepsia. *N Engl J Med* 1998; **26**: 1875–81.

19 Drumm B, Perez Perez GI, Blaser MJ, Sherman PM. Intrafamilial clustering of *Helicobacter pylori* infection. *N Engl J Med* 1990; **322**: 359–63.

20 Chey WD, Spybrook M, Carpenter S *et al.* Prolonged effect of omeprazole on the ^{14}C-urea breath test. *Am J Gastroenterol* 1996; **91**: 89–92.

21 Loy CT Irwig LM, Katelaris PH, Talley NJ. Do commercial serological kits for *H. pylori* infection differ in accuracy? A meta-analysis. *Am J Gastroenterol* 1996; **91** (6): 1138–44.

22 Chiba N, Rao BV, Rademaker JW, Hunt RH. Meta-analysis of the efficacy of antibiotic therapy in eradicating *Helicobacter pylori*. *Am J Gastroenterol* 1992; **87** (12): 1716–27.

23 Unge P, Berstad A. Pooled analysis of anti-*Helicobacter pylori* treatment regimens. *Scand J Gastroenterol* 1996; **31** (220): 27–40.

24 Taylor JL, Zagari M, Murphy K, Freston JW. Pharmacoeconomic comparison of treatments for the eradication of *Helicobacter pylori*. *Arch Intern Med* 1997; **157**: 87–97.

25 Crowe JP, Wilkinson SP, Bate CM, Willoughby CP, Peers EM, Richardson PDI. Symptom relief and duodenal ulcer healing with omeprazole or cimetidine. *Aliment Pharmacol Ther* 1989; **3**: 83–91.

4 Gastric cancer

Michael Bramble

Key Points

- There are 10 000 deaths per year from gastric cancer in the UK.
- In its early stages, gastric cancer has no diagnostic features.
- Age of the patient is an important determinant of risk.
- Overall 5-year survival rate is 30%, but for early gastric cancer it exceeds 90%.

Background

The aetiology of gastric cancer is multifactorial and has long been known to be associated with poor living conditions and poor diet, particularly low vitamin C intake [1]. Gastric atrophy and the associated intestinal metaplasia have also been a recognized risk factor for the intestinal type of cancer for many years [2], including atrophy associated with pernicious anaemia [3]. There is now strong evidence that *Helicobacter pylori* infection is a significant risk factor for the development of gastric cancer although the absolute risk is small [4–6]. The relative risk is greatest in younger *H. pylori*-infected patients [7] and those possessing the strain of *H. pylori* positive for the cytotoxin-associated gene *CagA* [8]. Patients with this strain are more likely to develop a pangastritis leading to hypochlorhydria, atrophic gastritis and intestinal metaplasia which are precancerous conditions [9]. Patients with pangastritis also have lower levels of vitamin C in the stomach as a result of lower secretion [10], thus linking previous knowledge about the importance of this vitamin to *H. pylori* infection. However, it should be recognized that *H. pylori* is only one small factor in the development of gastric cancer and the vast majority of patients with this organism will not develop the condition [11]. The rising incidence of adenocarcinoma at the cardia has not been fully explained but may be related to the rising incidence of gastro-oesophageal reflux disease [12].

The extent of the problem

Gastric cancer is a disease that is rare under the age of 40 years and affects men more than women, with an overall incidence of 10–20 per 100 000 population. Although the incidence is slowly declining in the USA and western Europe it remains the fourth commonest malignancy among men [13]. The decline is due to a decrease in the 'intestinal' type of adenocarcinoma affecting the antrum and corpus of the stomach [14]. However, there has been a 10-fold increase in the incidence of adenocarcinoma of the cardia [15], probably secondary to Barrett's or columnar lined oesophagus resulting from long-standing gastro-oesophageal reflux. This type of carcinoma is usually referred to as 'diffuse' type and occurs more commonly in younger people with a worse prognosis [16]. In the UK there are just under 10 000 deaths per annum from gastric cancer [17] and the incidence increases rapidly through the seventh and eighth decades of life [17]. The average general practice will see one case a year.

Adenocarcinoma of the cardia is usually of the diffuse type and the rising incidence may be secondary to the increasing prevalence of Barrett's oesophagus secondary to gastro-oesophageal reflux disease [18]. The risk of developing adenocarcinoma in Barrett's oesophagus is between 35 and 125 times greater than in an age-matched population [19]. Although most gastroenterologists screen for adenocarcinoma of the oesophagus in patients with Barrett's oesophagus, the frequency varies from 1 to 3 years [20]. Few patients present with early disease and so the prognosis remains dismal [13]. If gastric cancer is detected early then surgery offers worthwhile remission, or even cure [21]. Increasing general practitioner access to gastroscopy has not yet resulted in an increased detection rate for the earlier stages of the disease [22].

Presentation, diagnosis and investigation

Patients presenting with advanced disease usually have one or more 'alarm' symptoms including: (i) weight loss; (ii) dysphagia; and (iii) anaemia. Patients with early stage disease have benign symptoms [23] and so age alone determines the need to investigate late-onset dyspepsia by gastroscopy.

Clinical diagnosis and investigations

The clinical diagnosis is usually made at gastroscopy and biopsies obtained to confirm the endoscopic appearance [24]. Although multiple biopsies are recommended, even this policy may fail to detect malignant change in an otherwise benign-looking gastric ulcer, particularly if the patient has been on acid-suppression therapy prior to gastroscopy [25]. Further investigation by ultrasound and computed tomography will enable the clinician to determine whether the tumour is operable as this offers the only chance of cure in early stage disease [21].

Patients of any age with one or more of these symptoms should have an urgent gastroscopy [24], although it should be stated that surgical 'cure' is unlikely once worrying symptoms develop. Urgent gastroscopy (or barium meal) is mandatory for these patients [24]. Consider also the re-investigation of patients over the age of 40–45 years who present with further dyspepsia and who have had a previous normal gastroscopy [22]. All new-onset dyspepsia should be investigated in this age group, even if symptoms sound benign [23]. One risk of acid-suppression therapy prior to gastroscopy is a delay in the diagnosis of cancer [22,26]. H_2-receptor antagonists have the ability to mask both the symptoms and appearance of gastric cancer [27] and the advent of proton pump inhibitors has exacerbated this problem [25].

Staging of gastric cancer

Gastric cancer is staged according to the TNM (tumour, node, metastasis) classification of tumours [28], but this is a pathological staging classification and the exact stage will often not be known prior to surgery. Early gastric cancer is the description used when the tumour is confined to the mucosa, whilst stage I disease refers to the penetration of tumour into the submucosa (including localized lymph nodes close to the lesion). Both stages are potentially curable by surgery. Later stages II, III and IV are unlikely to be cured by surgery.

Management

Management is highly dependent on the stage of the disease at presentation. Supportive treatment is appropriate for many elderly patients with advanced disease. Good palliation can be obtained from surgery although relief is often transient [29].

Metallic stents provide excellent palliation from dysphagia [30] and are now being used for distal gastric obstruction in patients previously referred to surgery for a non-curative operation.

Good communication between primary and secondary care will ensure that patients who will benefit from palliative treatment such as stenting are identified and jointly managed.

Quality of life is paramount and can be evaluated by questionnaires. Analgesia, antiemetics, diet, haematinics and regular blood transfusion may all be useful in improving quality of life for patients with advanced disease. Surgery remains the cornerstone of treatment for patients with potentially curable disease. Results for early gastric cancer and stage I disease are very much better than those for later stage disease [21] but more radical surgery confers no survival advantage [24].

The overall prognosis is highly dependent on diagnosing early stage disease when symptoms are benign [23] and this should be the main goal of primary care management.

Follow-up and prognosis

Prognosis is determined by many factors including tumour differentiation, lymph node spread and the presence or absence of distal metastases. Chemotherapy offers little advantage if surgical resection is adequate [31]. Follow-up is important to detect problems that might arise as the result of surgery but very few patients will require further intervention. Overall, only about 30% of patients will survive 5 years [24] but this figure does hide the fact that patients with early gastric cancer have a 5-year survival rate in excess of 90% [21].

Screening and prevention

In the UK and most of western Europe, whole population screening for gastric cancer would not be cost-effective although the same may not be true for patients known to be at risk of oesophageal adenocarcinoma as a result of having Barrett's oesophagus.

References

1 O'Toole P, Lombard M. Vitamin C and gastric cancer: supplements for some or fruit for all? *Gut* 1996; **39**: 345–7.

2 Morson BC. Carcinoma arising from areas of intestinal metaplasia in the gastric mucosa. *Br J Cancer* 1955; **9**: 377–85.

3 Brinton I, Grindley G, Hrubec Z, Hoover R, Fraumeni JF. Cancer risk following pernicious anaemia. *Br J Cancer* 1989; **59**: 810–13.

4 The EUROGAST Study Group. An international association between *Helicobacter pylori* infection and gastric cancer. *Lancet* 1993; **341**: 1359–62.

5 Parsonnet J, Friedman GD, Vandersteen DP *et al.* Helicobacter infection and the risk of gastric cancer. *N Engl J Med* 1991; **325**: 1127–31.

6 Forman D, Newell DG, Fullerton F, Yarnell JW, Stacey AR, Wald N, Sitas F. Association between infection with *Helicobacter pylori* and the risk of gastric cancer: evidence from a prospective investigation. *BMJ* 1991; **302**: 1302–5.

7 Huang JQ, Sridhar S, Chen Y, Hunt RH. Meta-analysis of the relationship between *Helicobacter pylori* seropositivity and gastric cancer. *Gastroenterology* 1998; **114**: 1169–79.

8 Parsonnet AJ, Friedman GD, Orenstriech N, Vogelman H. Risk for gastric cancer in people with Cag A negative *Helicobacter pylori* infection. *Gut* 1997; **40**: 297–301.

9 Sipponen P, Kekki M, Haapakoski J, Ihamaki T, Siurali M. Gastric cancer risk in chronic atrophic gastritis: statistical calculations of cross sectional data. *Int J Cancer* 1985; **35**: 173–7.

10 Zhang ZW, Patchett SE, Perrett D, Katelaris PH, Domizio P, Farthing MJG. The relation between gastric vitamin C concentrations, mucosal histology and Cag A seropositivity in the human stomach. *Gut* 1998; **43**: 322–6.

11 Fuchs CS, Mayer RJ. Gastric carcinoma. *N Engl J Med* 1995; **333**: 32–41.

12 Lagergren J, Bergstrom R, Lindgren A, Nyren O. Symptomatic gastro-esophageal reflux as a risk factor for esophageal adenocarcinoma. *N Engl J Med* 1999; **340**: 825–31.

13 Thompson GB, van Heerden JA, Saar MG. Adenocarcinoma of the stomach: are we making progress? *Lancet* 1993; **342**: 713–18.

14 Craanen ME, Dekker W, Blok P, Ferwerda J, Tytgat GN. Time trends in gastric carcinoma: changing patterns of type and location. *Am J Gastroenterol* 1992; **87**: 572–9.

15 Pera M, Cameron AJ, Trastek VF *et al.* Increasing incidence of adenocarcinoma of the oesophagus and oesophagogastric junction. *Gastroenterology* 1993; **104**: 510–13.

16 Lauren PA, Nevalainen JT. Epidemiology of intestinal and diffuse types of gastric carcinoma: a time trend study in Finland with comparison between studies from high and low risk areas. *Cancer* 1993; **712**: 926–33.

17 Lambert R. The role of endoscopy in the prevention of esophagogastric cancer. *Endoscopy* 1999; **31**: 180–99.

18 Spechler S. Barrett's oesophagus. *Semin Oncol* 1994; **21**: 431–7.

19 Provenzale D, Kemp JA, Arora S, Wong JB. A guide for surveillance of patients with Barrett's esophagus. *Am J Gastroenterol* 1994; **89**: 670–80.

20 Ackroyd R, Wakefield SE, Williams JL, Stoddart CJ, Reed MW. Surveillance of Barrett's esophagus: a need for guidelines? *Dis Esophagus* 1997; **10**: 185–9.

21 Sue-Ling HM, Johnson D, Martin IG *et al.* Gastric cancer: a curable disease in Britain. *BMJ* 1993; **307**: 591–6.

22 Suvakovic Z, Bramble MG, Jones R, Wilson C, Idle N, Ryott J. Improving the detection rate of early gastric cancer requires more than open access gastroscopy. A five-year study. *Gut* 1997; **41**: 308–13.

23 Fielding JWL, Ellis DJ, Jones BG *et al.* Natural history of 'early' gastric cancer: results of a ten year regional survey. *BMJ* 1980; **281**: 965–7.

24 Cuschieri A, Fayers P, Fielding J *et al.* Postoperative morbidity and mortality after D1 and D2 resections for gastric cancer: preliminary results of the MRC randomised controlled surgical trial. *Lancet* 1996; **347**: 995–9.

4

24 Axon ATR, Bell GD, Jones R, Quine A, McCloy R. Guidelines on appropriate indications for upper gastrointestinal endoscopy. *BMJ* 1995; **310**: 853–6.

25 Wayman J, Hayes N, Biggin CS, Karat D, Raimes SA, Griffin SM. Response of early gastric cancer to proton pump inhibitors. *N Engl J Med* 1998; **338**: 1924–5.

26 Martin IG, Young S, Sue-Ling HM, Johnson D. Delays in the diagnosis of oesophagogastric cancer: a consecutive case series. *BMJ* 1997; **314**: 467–71.

27 Taylor RH, Lovell D, Menzies-Gow N, LaBrooy SJ, Misiewicz JJ. Misleading response of malignant ulcers to cimetidine. *Lancet* 1978; **i**: 686–8.

28 Kennedy BJ. TNM classification for stomach cancer. *Cancer* 1970; **26**: 971–83.

29 Ekbom GA, Gleysteen JJ. Gastric malignancy: resection for palliation. *Surgery* 1980; **88**: 476–81.

30 Knyrim K, Wagner HJ, Bethge N, Keymling M, Valik N. A controlled trial of an expansile metal stent for palliation of esophageal obstruction due to inoperable cancer. *N Engl J Med* 1993; **329**: 1302–7.

31 Lise M, Nitti D, Marchet A *et al.* Prognostic factors in resectable gastric cancer: results or EORTC study no. 40813 on FAM adjuvant chemotherapy. *Ann Surg Oncol* 1995; **2**: 495–501.

4

5 Gallbladder and biliary problems

Pali Hungin

Key Points

- Gallstones affect 20% of the population.
- 60% of gallstones are symptomless.
- Gallstones may present acutely with colic or cholecystitis, or chronically with recurrent upper abdominal pain and dyspepsia.
- 75% of cholecystectomies are now laparoscopic.
- Dissolution therapy and lithotripsy are now rarely used.

Introduction

Gallstones affect up to a fifth of the population and 50 000 cholecystectomies are carried out every year in the UK. The male/female ratio is 0.4 : 1 mainly in the 45–64 age group [1] with a preponderance in the multiparous and obese.

There are essentially two types of gallstones: cholesterol stones and pigment stones. Cholesterol stones constitute 70% of the total and are the result of the secretion of cholesteraemic bile. Pigment stones are linked with an excess of unprecipated bilirubin. Softer and more friable stones, usually of the pigment sort, are more associated with infections of the biliary tree.

The commonest manifestation of gallstones is either biliary colic or cholecystitis. Up to 60% of gallstones are symptomless but the impaction of a stone in the gallbladder neck can cause inflammation and severe pain. The symptoms may be short lasting (less than an hour) if the stone passes spontaneously but biliary obstruction and jaundice can occur if the stone lodges in the common bile duct. Bacterial infection from stones in the common bile duct results in cholangitis, a potentially life-threatening illness, and, less commonly, liver abscess formation.

Biliary colic, a spasmodic upper abdominal pain, is due to the impaction of one or more stones in the gallbladder neck, in the common bile duct or close to the ampulla. The passage of the stone beyond the obstruction is linked with relief of symptoms.

Management of cholecystitis

Acute cholecystitis

This usually presents with pain of sudden onset, in the epigastrium, radiating to the back, sometimes with vomiting. Episodes can be as short as 15 min but symptoms may last up to 24 h, longer-lasting episodes with fever indicating the possibility of cholangitis. Management is usually conservative with analgesics (e.g. injected pethidine) and antispasmodics. Broad-spectrum antibiotics (e.g. amoxicillin or cephalosporins) are advocated [1] and failure to respond usually results in hospital admission.

Following confirmation of the diagnosis cholecystectomy is now increasingly performed within a few days of the episode. Contrary to advice 10–15 years ago, evidence suggests that early cholecystectomy, rather than a few months later, is associated with a high success rate and fewer complications [2]. About 10% of patients with acute cholecystitis have stones in the common bile duct and preoperative endoscopic retrograde cholangiopancreatography (ERCP) or peroperative cholangiography is required. Abnormal liver function tests should alert the clinician to this possibility.

Chronic cholecystitis

This is more common than acute cholecystitis and is due to chronic inflammation and thickening of the gallbladder wall. It usually develops insidiously but can follow an acute attack of cholecystitis. The condition usually manifests as right hypochondrial or epigastric pain, radiating to the back or scapula. Non-specific symptoms such as abdominal discomfort, flatulence and intolerance of fatty foods may constitute the only symptoms.

The treatment of choice is cholecystectomy. This leads to complete abolition of symptoms providing they were due to the gallbladder. As the symptoms of chronic cholecystitis frequently overlap with dyspepsia, gastro-oesophageal reflux and colonic problems due to functional disorders, diagnostic certainty is a problem. Many surgeons resort to a routine preoperative gastroscopy in an attempt to exclude other problems but this approach has not been proven to be conclusively effective.

A conservative approach, involving weight reduction and a low-fat diet, may help limit symptoms. Dissolution therapy may be a possibility for some (see below).

Common bile duct stones

Most of these originate from the gallbladder, with 10% of those with gallstones also having duct stones. The usual symptoms are colicky, severe pain lasting for hours, often with vomiting, sometimes with jaundice, pale faeces and dark urine. Similar symptoms can be caused by carcinoma of the head of pancreas, biliary ampulla or bile duct and by acute viral or alcoholic hepatitis.

Endoscopic retrograde cholangiopancreatography is increasingly commonly used for the diagnosis and management of common bile duct stones. This enables such stones to be visualized and removed with endoscopically introduced retrieval instruments following a sphincteroctomy. In patients not suitable for operation this technique can also be used to distend the sphincter of Oddi to facilitate the escape of stones.

Silent gallstones

Sixty per cent of patients with gallstones experience no symptoms. They are at little risk of developing complications, the yearly risk of developing symptoms being 1–4%. No action is necessary unless the patient is young, in which case there is the increasing possibility of problems with age. Diabetic patients are more prone to developing cholecystitis. Any possible gains from a cholecystectomy have to be weighed against the possibility of complications and postoperative side effects such as diarrhoea.

Post-cholecystectomy problems

The following problems can occur after cholecystectomy:
1 Increase in stool frequency or diarrhoea (up to 10% of patients).
2 Bile duct injury during operation (0.5%).
3 Retained or recurrent stones.
4 Ampullary stenosis.

Medical management of gallstones

This is essentially for patients not considered appropriate for surgical management and consists of either drugs that dissolve gallstones or physical methods, such as extra-corporeal shock wave lithotripsy. Since the advent of laparoscopic cholecystectomy these are now rarely used. An evaluation of the effectiveness of dissolution therapy [3] reported in the Cochrane Library indicates that success rates are better with higher doses and in patients with smaller stones (less than 10 mm diameter). Dissolution therapy is likely to be suitable for no more than 15% of patients who have radiolucent stones within a functioning gallbladder [3]. A major problem is the chance of recurrence of stones.

5

Cholecystectomy: open or laparoscopic?

Over 75% of cholecystectomies are now carried out laparoscopically. A major advantage is that recovery is faster than from an open operation and most patients can be discharged within 48 h. Contrary to popular belief, the procedure actually requires four access points rather than only one but there are few contraindications, advanced pregnancy and coagulation disorders being the chief ones.

The commonest complication of laparoscopic cholecystectomy is bile leak during the operation from injury to the ductal system, usually the common bile duct. Laparoscopic cholecystectomy is also suitable for patients with acute cholecystitis although this has a higher rate of conversion to an open procedure. Overall data [4] indicate that laparscopic cholecystectomy has a lower mortality (8–9 per 10 000) than an open operation and is suitable for a wider group of patients. A major factor in the safety and rates of 'conversion' to an open operation is the level of the surgeon's expertise. Recognized training and expertise are prerequisites for those using this technique. Rates of conversion to an open operation vary between institutions but are around 5% and the risk of common bile duct injury is around 0.5% [4].

References

1 Summerfield JA. Gall-stones: Clinical features and medical management. In: Misiewicz JJ, Pounder RE, Venables CW, eds. *Diseases of the Gut and Pancreas.* Oxford: Blackwell Scientific Publications, 1994.
2 McArthur P, Cuschieri A, Sells RA, Shields R. Controlled clinical trial comparing early with interval cholecystectomy for acute cholecystitis. *Br J Surg* 1975; **62**: 850–2.

3 May GR, Sutherland LR, Shaffer EA. Efficacy of bile acid therapy for gallstone dissolution: a meta-analysis of randomised trials. *Aliment Pharmacol Ther* 1993; **7**: 139–48.

4 Shea JA, Healey MJ, Berlin JA *et al.* Mortality and complications associated with laparoscopic cholecystectomy: a meta-analysis. *Ann Surg* 1996; **224**: 609–20.

5

6 Liver problems

Michael Bramble

Key Points

• Symptoms of liver disease are often non-specific.
• Initial investigations comprise liver function tests, immunology and ultrasound scan of the liver.
• The important causes of liver disease are alcohol, chronic viral hepatitis, primary biliary cirrhosis and autoimmune disorders.
• Most patients need specialist management. Abstinence from alcohol is the only treatment for pre-cirrhotic alcoholic liver disease.

Background

Alcoholic liver disease

Alcohol is the most significant cause of liver disease in the UK and is the most important risk factor for the development of cirrhosis [1]. Deaths from alcoholic liver disease are increasing in some countries [2] although overall alcohol consumption is not increasing [3]. There are marked geographical variations in alcohol consumption, which may explain this discrepancy [3]. Fatty infiltration of the liver (steato-hepatitis) is the usual forerunner to developing cirrhosis and patients with this stage of alcoholic liver disease should be warned about progression to cirrhosis with continuing alcohol consumption [4]. Many patients simply present with end-stage cirrhosis and come to light as a consequence of developing complications such as ascites or variceal bleeding.

Non-alcoholic fatty liver does not progress to cirrhosis and patients discovered to have this condition on ultrasonography should be reassured [5].

Autoimmune liver disease

Autoimmune hepatitis is a persisting inflammatory process within the liver, the cause of which is unknown. A few patients show false-positive results for hepatitis C and approximately 10% of patients with hepatitis C have autoantibodies [6]. Autoantibodies are necessary for the diagnosis but as with other autoimmune diseases they are not 100% specific. Females are affected more than males and two-thirds have autoantibodies to smooth muscle and antinuclear factor [7]. Three different types of autoimmune hepatitis are recognized, based on other factors including the presence of other autoantibodies. Immunoglogulin levels, particularly IgG, are increased. Untreated, such patients go on to develop end-stage cirrhosis.

Primary biliary cirrhosis

This term is now a misnomer as the majority of patients present with abnormal liver function tests rather than with established cirrhosis [8]. The cause remains unknown. The condition predominantly affects females and antimitochrondrial antibodies (antibodies to pyruvate dehydrogenase complex) at a titre greater than 1 in 20 are found in 96% of patients with this disease. Serum IgM and IgG are usually increased but this may be in association with a general increase in immunoglogulin levels. Liver histology shows progressive destruction of the small intrahepatic bile ducts and portal inflammatory infiltrate which eventually leads to fibrosis or cirrhosis. The damage is often not uniform and prognosis is only partly determined by the histological stage [9].

Chronic viral hepatitis

Hepatitis B

Hepatitis B is a 42-nm DNA virus with an incubation period of 28–180 days. Infection via blood transfusion is now very rare unless this takes place in a country with no screening of transfused blood. The majority of patients are now infected by use of unsterilized needles (intravenous drug abusers) or through sexual contact. Approximately 20% of infected individuals go on to develop chronic hepatitis. Liver histology varies from patients with no detectable histological abnormality through to active hepatitis, portal fibrosis and eventually end-stage cirrhosis. Hepatitis B is a risk factor for the development of a primary hepatoma even in the absence of cirrhosis [10].

Hepatitis C

This virus was discovered by molecular cloning in 1989 [11] and is now known to be the main cause of non-A, non-B, post-transfusion hepatitis. In North America there are an estimated four million carriers and cirrhosis secondary to hepatitis C is now the leading indication for liver transplantation. The number of patients with hepatitis C is likely to increase significantly over the next 20 years [12]. Transmission is unknown for a large proportion of patients with this disease [13] but sexual transmission is thought to be one possibility [14].

The extent of the problem

Alcoholic liver disease

6

In broad terms alcoholic liver disease is far more common than other forms of chronic hepatitis in many populations. The true prevalence of alcoholic liver disease is not known and there are marked differences both within and between countries [1–3]. Genetic factors are important in determining susceptibility to liver injury from alcohol excess. The majority of patients ingesting levels of alcohol over and above the designated safe limits will not develop cirrhosis [4].

Autoimmune liver disease

This disorder is characterized by finding positive autoantibodies in the serum, predominantly antinuclear factor (ANF) and smooth muscle antibody (SMA). The incidence varies from country to country but approximately one-third are men [6] and autoimmunity accounts for 20% of all chronic hepatitis in the *developed* world [15]. There is a known association with other autoimmune diseases.

Primary biliary cirrhosis

The incidence of primary biliary cirrhosis (PBC) varies geographically. In the UK the highest incidence is in the north-east of England [16] with a reported prevalence of 128 per million in 1987. Elsewhere the prevalence varies between 20 and 240 per million with an annual incidence between 4 and 30 per million [17]. The condition may present at any age and many patients are discovered by chance when liver function tests are carried out.

Chronic viral hepatitis

Hepatitis B

World-wide this is a common cause of chronic hepatitis, cirrhosis and hepatoma with an estimated 350 million carriers. In the UK the disease is uncommon and affects only 1–2% of the population. Chronic hepatitis is common following acute infection and affects 10–20% of people. Symptom-free carriage rate is also about 1% and more common in residents born outside the UK [18].

Hepatitis C

The prevalence in the UK is unknown but a carriage rate of 0.9% has been recorded from an inner-city health district [18]. The majority of people infected become chronic carriers (75–85%) and disease progression to cirrhosis is slow, determined by many factors including infection in patients over the age of 50 years, male sex and excess alcohol consumption [9]. World-wide the prevalence varies from 1–15% [20,21] but in the USA the majority of infections is linked to intravenous drug abuse [22].

Presentation and common symptoms

Many patients with liver disease will have no symptoms or only non-specific symptoms such as fatigue. This applies to the majority of patients with autoimmune hepatitis, chronic viral hepatitis and PBC. The diagnosis is often revealed only after liver function tests have been performed.

Alcoholic liver disease

Generally speaking patients with alcoholic liver disease tend to present late, when symptoms and clinical signs are well established. These include cirrhosis with jaundice, ascites, peripheral oedema, bruising and/ or early encephalopathy.

Autoimmune liver disease

Patients with autoimmune hepatitis may present at any stage, ranging from those with asymptomatic disease through to those presenting with acute hepatitis (40%) including fulminating hepatitis or chronic liver failure in a previously well person. Painless jaundice, oedema, ascites and variceal bleeding are manifestations of advanced disease.

Primary biliary cirrhosis

Symptoms are often debilitating due to itch and/or fatigue. The diagnosis is usually triggered by finding cholestatic liver function tests in a middle-aged or elderly woman with non-specific symptoms. The disease is divided into four stages ranging from symptomless patients with normal liver tests through to those with end-stage cirrhosis [23,24].

Chronic viral hepatitis

Hepatitis B

Symptoms are dependent on the stage of the disease in common with other types of chronic hepatitis. In the pre-cirrhotic phase many patients are asymptomatic or complain only of non-specific symptoms such as fatigue.

Hepatitis C

The acute infection is usually associated with little in the way of symptoms and many patients known to carry the hepatitis C virus have no apparent risk factors. The majority of people infected become chronic carriers but progression to cirrhosis is extremely slow [19].

Clinical diagnosis and investigations

Alcoholic liver disease

Although the diagnosis may be obvious, patients may hide alcohol dependence from their family and their general practitioner. Suspicions are often aroused only by a persistent finding of an elevated γ-glutamyltransferase (γGT) associated with macrocytosis. A random blood alcohol or urine alcohol will often surprise the person requesting it by its magnitude. Investigation by ultrasound scan of the liver usually shows fatty infiltration but may include more serious complications such as cirrhosis and portal hypertension.

Autoimmune liver disease

Diagnosis is usually made on liver biopsy but many patients will already have cirrhosis at this time [24]. Liver function tests characteristically show elevation of SGOT and SGPT with less or no change in alkaline phosphatase and γGT. Autoantibodies are usually positive for smooth muscle or ANF. DNA antibodies are positive in patients with systemic lupus. In PBC the picture is one of elevated alkaline phosphatase and γGT associated with positive antimitochondrial antibodies.

Primary biliary cirrhosis

Diagnosis is usually triggered by finding cholestatic liver function test in a middle-aged or elderly woman with non-specific symptoms [25]. Antimitochondrial antibodies are positive at a titre greater than 1 in 20. Liver biopsy is useful in staging the disease in young adults, but may not be necessary in older patients with a typical biochemical profile of raised alkaline phosphatase and γGT with a strongly positive antimitochondrial antibody titre. An ultrasound scan of the liver can confirm portal hypertension and exclude anatomical causes for the abnormal liver function tests.

Chronic viral hepatitis

Hepatitis B

Persistently abnormal liver function tests associated with a positive hepatitis B surface antigen (HBsAg) indicate that the patient has chronic hepatitis B although patients with this picture will be of low infectivity only if the core antibody is positive. The structurally related e antigen (HBeAg) indicates that the patient is highly infectious.

Hepatitis B virus DNA (HBV DNA) can be detected in patients with active viral replication and can be used to monitor the effect of treatment with interferon alfa. A positive response to treatment involves resolution of abnormal liver function tests associated with loss of HBeAg and HBV DNA. Approximately 40% of patients will respond in this way [27]. Hepatitis B is a major risk factor for hepatocellular carcinoma once cirrhosis has developed. Monitoring of the serum alfa-fetoprotein levels should be part of the regular testing in this group of patients.

Hepatitis C

Diagnosis is made by checking the patient's serum for HBV antibodies and excluding other causes of persistently abnormal liver function tests. An increasing number of patients are referred from the blood transfusion service where routine screening picks up patients with no previous history of hepatitis. There is poor correlation between liver function tests and the degree of viral liver damage [20] and liver biopsy should be carried out in all patients if treatment is contemplated because cirrhosis reduces the chances of responding to interferon alfa [28].

6

Management

Most patients with persistently abnormal liver function tests should have a detailed history taken to exclude alcohol and drug-related causes for the abnormality. A full hepatitis and autoantibody screen will detect those patients with chronic viral hepatitis and autoimmune disease. All patients should have an ultrasound scan to determine whether the liver is anatomically normal. Many will need referral to hospital for further investigations including liver biopsy.

Autoimmune liver disease

Oral corticosteroids remain the mainstay of treatment for patients with autoimmune hepatitis [29] although the liver biopsy appearances are a more reliable indicator of the need for treatment than liver function tests. Current treatment regimens have a failure rate of approximately 13% [30]. High-dose oral corticosteroids (1 mg/kg/day) are used to establish a remission and the dose is tailed down to a maintenance dose of 5–10 mg daily depending on liver function tests. Patients requiring high-dose steroids (>10 mg/day) to control their disease should be started on azathioprine as a steroid-sparing agent [30]. Treatment is often for life, but a trial of treatment withdrawal is justified after 5 years for patients with mild disease. A significant number of patients do relapse and close follow-up is required [31].

Primary biliary cirrhosis

Treatment is directed towards controlling symptoms and complications such as osteomalacia secondary to malabsorption of the fat-soluble vitamins (A, D and K). Itching may respond to cholestyramine or opioid antagonists but the lethargy associated with PBC is harder to treat [8]. The majority of patients are treated with ursodeoxycholic acid. This improves liver function tests but probably does not affect progression to cirrhosis [8]. Disease progression is slow and many patients will have no major clinical deterioration over several years [23]. Transplantation is the treatment of choice as the development of symptoms correlates with prognosis and mortality [32]. The disease can recur in the transplanted liver but this is not a contraindication to operation as the disease progression is slow [33].

6 Chronic viral hepatitis

Hepatitis B

The currently recommended therapy for chronic hepatitis B is interferon alfa at a high dose for 6 months [28]. The treatment is expensive and causes significant side effects. Oral lamivudine, which results in inhibition of HBV DNA, is also useful although relapse is almost universal when treatment is stopped. New therapies are in the process of development [34].

Hepatitis C

Longer courses of interferon alfa are required to treat chronic hepatitis (12–18 months) and response is much more variable depending on the viral genome. The weekly dose is lower than in hepatitis B but still associated with many side effects.

Treatment of chronic hepatitis C is still evolving but therapy is offered to those with moderate disease [35]. The only effective treatment is interferon alfa. The sustained response rate is only 20%. Newer regimens incorporating oral ribavirin seem to be more effective, with a doubling of the sustained response rate in suitable patients [36].

Alcoholic liver disease

The only effective treatment for pre-cirrhotic disease is for the patient to abstain from alcohol. Patients who have already developed cirrhosis may require treatment directed towards control of ascites (diuretics) and portal hypertension (beta-blockers). Alcoholic cirrhosis is now the commonest reason for liver transplantation in the USA and is of increasing importance in the UK and Europe [37].

Follow-up and prognosis

Alcoholic liver disease

Patients with decompensated liver disease will require hospital follow-up, in order to effectively manage many of the complications of end-stage liver disease. This applies to other forms of chronic liver disease, in which end-stage cirrhosis results in a number of problems such as portal hypertension, encephalopathy and variceal bleeding.

Primary biliary cirrhosis

Hepatic function is maintained for a very long period of time and falls only in the late stages. Serum bilirubin is a good prognostic marker as estimated survival is less than 18 months once the bilirubin level has reached 170 µmol/l [32]. Liver transplantation is the treatment of choice once this stage has been reached with the 5-year survival rate excellent at 80%.

Chronic viral hepatitis

Patients with chronic HBV or HCV infection require referral to hospital for a detailed evaluation of liver function and disease activity. Patients with inactive disease can be followed up in primary care and those with well-compensated cirrhosis can be cared for in general practice as the disease progression is usually very slow. However, a significant number of patients have persistently abnormal liver function tests due to chronic hepatitis. Some of these will develop cirrhosis and hepatocellular carcinoma [10]. Patients with chronic viral hepatitis should be strongly advised to avoid alcohol as this increases the risks associated with chronic viral hepatitis.

Screening and prevention

The important message is that liver disease is often occult and may

6

be the reason for a non-specific deterioration in the patient's health. Macrocytosis on blood film may give a clue to the aetiology being alcohol related, but in most cases the patient will be complaining only of vague symptoms such as fatigue, arthralgia or itching. Many patients will be picked up coincidentally when tests are arranged to investigate such symptoms.

References

1 Corrao G, Zambon A, Torchio P, La Vecchia C, di Orio F. Attributable risk for symptomatic liver cirrhosis in Italy. Collaborative group for the study of liver diseases in Italy. *J Hepatol* 1998; **28**: 608–14.
2 Chick J. Evidence suggesting increasing health damage in Scotland related to alcohol. *Health Bull (Edinb)* 1997; **55**: 134–9.
3 Adang RP, Wensing JW, Stockbrugger RW. Alcohol consumption and alcohol-related liver disease in The Netherlands. *Scand J Gastroenterol Suppl* 1998; **225**: 70–4.
4 Teli MR, Day CP, Burt AD, Bennett MK, James OF. Determinants of progression to cirrhosis or fibrosis in pure alcoholic fatty liver. *Lancet* 1995; **346**: 987–90.
5 Teli MR, James OF, Burt AD, Bennett MK, Day CP. The natural history of nonalcoholic fatty liver: a follow up study. *Hepatology* 1995; **22**: 1714–19.
6 Meyer Z, Buschenfelde KH, Lohse AW. Autoimmune hepatitis. *N Engl J Med* 1995; **333**: 1004–5.
7 Lohse AW, Gerken G, Mohr H *et al.* Distinction between autoimmune liver diseases and viral hepatitis: clinical and serological characteristics in 859 patients. *Z Gastroenterol* 1995; **33**: 527–33.
8 Neuberger, J. Primary biliary cirrhosis. *Lancet* 1997; **350**: 875–9.
9 Garrido MC, Hubscher SG. Accuracy of staging in primary biliary cirrhosis. *J Clin Pathol* 1996; **49**: 556–9.
10 Viola LA, Barrison IG, Coleman JC *et al.* Natural history of liver disease in chronic hepatitis B surface antigen carriers. Survey of 100 patients from Great Britain. *Lancet* 1981; **ii**: 1156–9.
11 Choo Q-L, Kuo G, Weiner AJ *et al.* Isolation of cDNA clone derived from a blood borne non-A, non-B viral hepatitis genome. *Science* 1989; **244**: 359–62.
12 National Institutes of Health consensus development conference panel statement. Management of hepatitis C. *Hepatology* 1997; **26**: 2S–10S.
13 Heintges T, Wands JR. Hepatitis C virus: epidemiology and transmission. *Hepatology* 1997; **26**: 521–6.
14 Salleras L, Bruguera M, Vidal J *et al.* Importance of sexual transmission of hepatitis C in seropositive pregnant women: a case control study. *J Med Virol* 1997; **52**: 164–7.
15 Holdstock G, Rassam S, Millward-Sadler GH, Wright R. Different aetiology of chronic hepatitis in UK and Iraq. *Liver* 1983; **3**: 2–7.
16 Myszor M, James O. The epidemiology of primary biliary cirrhosis in northern England: an increasingly common disease? *Q J Med* 1990; **75**: 377–85.
17 Metcalf J, Howel D, James O, Bhopal R. Primary biliary cirrhosis: epidemiology helping the clinician. *BMJ* 1996; **312**: 1181–2.

18 King R, Johnson PJ, White YS, Smith HM, Williams R. Frequency of asymptomatic hepatitis types B and C in an inner city community and relation to possible risk factors. *Q J Med* 1991; **80**: 641–9.

19 Poynard T, Bedossa P, Opolon P. Natural history of liver fibrosis progression in patients with chronic hepatitis C. *Lancet* 1997; **349**: 825–32.

20 Di Bosceglie AM. Hepatitis C. *Lancet* 1998; **351**: 351–5.

21 Sallie R, King R, Silva E, Tibbs C, Johnson P, Williams R. Community prevalence of hepatitis C viraemia: a polymerase chain reaction study, *J Med Virol* 1994; **43**: 111–14.

22 Conry-Cantilena C, Van Raden M, Gribble J *et al.* Routes of infestation, viraemia and liver disease in asymptomatic individuals with hepatitis C virus infection. *N Engl J Med* 1996; **334**: 1691–6.

23 Metcalf JV. Natural history of early primary biliary cirrhosis. *Lancet* 1996; **348**: 1399–402.

24 Sherlock S. The management of chronic hepatitis. *Curr Opin Gastroenterol* 1996; **12**: 217–23.

25 Mitchison HC, Lucey MR, Kelly PJ, Neuberger JM, Williams R, James OF. Symptom development and prognosis in primary biliary cirrhosis: a study in two centres. *Gastroenterology* 1990; **99**: 778–84.

26 Bennett WG, Inoue Y, Beck JR, Wong JB, Pauker SG, Davis GL. Estimates of the cost effectiveness of a single course of interferon-a2b in patients with histologically mild chronic hepatitis C. *Ann Intern Med* 1997; **127**: 855–65.

27 Niederau C, Meintges T, Lange S *et al.* Long-term follow-up of HBeAg-positive patients treated with interferon alfa for chronic hepatitis B. *N Engl J Med* 1996; **334**: 1422–7.

28 Hoofnagle J, DiBisceglie A. The treatment of chronic viral hepatitis. *New Engl J Med* 1997; **336**: 347–54.

29 Van den Berg AP. Autoimmune hepatitis: pathogenesis, diagnosis and treatment. *Scand J Gastroenterol Suppl* 1998; **225**: 66–9.

30 Johnson PJ, McFarlane IG, Williams R. Azathioprine for long-term maintenance of remission in autoimmune hepatitis. *N Engl J Med* 1995; **333**: 958–63.

31 Hegarty JE, Nouri Aria KT, Portmann B. Eddleston AL, Williams R. Relapse following treatment withdrawal in patients with autoimmune chronic active hepatitis. *Hepatology* 1983; **3**: 685–9.

32 Shapiro J, Smith H, Schaffner F. Serum bilirubin: a prognostic factor in primary biliary cirrhosis. *Gut* 1979; **20**: 137–40.

33 Neuberger J. Recurrence of primary biliary cirrhosis, primary sclerosing cholangitis and autoimmune hepatitis. *Liver Transpl Surg* 1995; **1**: 109–15.

34 Pianko S, McHutchinson J. Chronic hepatitis B: new therapies on the horizon? *Lancet* 1999; **354**: 1662–3.

35 Foster GR, Goldin RD, Main J, Murray-Lyon I, Hargreaves S, Thomas HC. Management of chronic viral hepatitis C; clinical audit of biopsy-based management algorithm. *BMJ* 1997; **315**: 453–8.

36 Reichard O, Norkrans G, Fryden A, Braconier JH, Sonnerborg A, Weiland O. Randomised, double-blind, placebo-controlled trial of interferon alpha 2b with and without ribavirin for chronic hepatitis C. *Lancet* 1998; **352**: 83–7.

37 Neuburger J. Transplantation for alcoholic liver disease: a perspective from Europe. *Liver Transpl Surg* 1998; **4**: S51–7.

6

7 Acute and chronic pancreatitis

Michael Bramble

ACUTE PANCREATITIS

Key Points

- Most causes of acute pancreatitis are associated with gallstones or alcohol abuse.
- Diagnosis is confirmed by a raised serum amylase or lipase.
- Initial treatment is supportive.
- Acute pancreatitis carries a mortality of 5–10%.

Aetiology and presentation

Acute pancreatitis is an inflammatory process which can also extend outside the pancreas in severe cases. The majority of cases (80–90%) are associated with gallstones or alcohol abuse [1]. The remaining 10% appear to have no obvious cause although recent work suggests that many may still be due to very small gallstones or biliary sludge [2]. The incidence varies with geographical location and correlates with the incidence of gallstones and alcohol abuse. Although most cases are mild and self limiting, severe cases remain a difficult management problem with a mortality of 5–10% [3].

Patients present clinically with a continuous but slowly worsening epigastric pain which has a boring quality to it and frequently radiates to the back. Admission to hospital is required due to the severity of the pain where diagnosis is confirmed by the finding of a raised serum amylase or lipase [4].

Management

Moderate or severe pancreatitis requires hospital admission for supportive therapy including intravenous fluids (the patient is kept nil by mouth) and parenteral analgesia, usually opiate based. If gallstones are suspected as the cause of acute pancreatitis, urgent endoscopic retrograde cholangiopancreatography (ERCP) with sphincterotomy and stone extraction will enhance recovery and reduce morbidity due to cholangitis [5].

Within primary care the most important aspect of management is to recognize the clinical presentation of acute pancreatitis and refer those with moderate or severe disease for further investigation and treatment. Patients should be warned, following an attack secondary to alcohol abuse, that further, possibly life-threatening attacks are likely if alcohol consumption continues. If the attack is secondary to gallstones, cholecystectomy is the preferred intervention whilst endoscopic clearance of the common bile duct will prevent further pancreatitis in the majority of patients [6,7].

CHRONIC PANCREATITIS

Key Points

- Presents with unexplained upper abdominal pain. Gastroscopy and ultrasound are often normal.
- Treatment is intended to counter the effects of pancreatic insufficiency and to relieve pain.

Aetiology and presentation

Although uncommon, chronic pancreatitis is difficult to diagnose in general practice and can be overlooked as a cause of unexplained upper abdominal pain. The condition may arise from frequent episodes of acute or subacute pancreatitis secondary to alcohol abuse. End-stage disease with exocrine insufficiency is recognizable with steatorrhoea as the predominant symptom. Approximately 50% of these patients go on to develop pancreatic endocrine insufficiency and insulin-dependent diabetes mellitus [8]. Many of these patients do not have a history of recurrent abdominal pain although a plain abdominal film may show pancreatic calcification.

More indolent disease is difficult to diagnose in primary care as the diagnosis often requires imaging techniques such as computed tomography (CT) scanning, ERCP or magnetic resonance cholangiopancreatography (MRCP), as well as indirect tests of pancreatic exocrine function. Routine blood tests are of little value and ultrasonography is relatively insensitive in the absence of pancreatic calcification. Many patients with milder forms of chronic pancreatitis are misdiagnosed because of previously normal investigations. The diagnosis should be considered as a possibility for patients who appear to have genuine and persistent upper abdominal pain (possibly radiating to the back), in whom gastroscopy and ultrasonography are normal.

Management

Patients with suspected pancreatic disease should be referred to hospital for further investigations. An accurate diagnosis may pose problems even in the hospital setting because some patients have no or only 'minimal' changes on ERCP [9]. Treatment of chronic pancreatitis is directed essentially towards control of the principal symptoms.

Pancreatic insufficiency

Those patients with steatorrhoea and weight loss due to exocrine insufficiency and resultant maldigestion benefit from pancreatic enzyme supplementation given with food. Acid suppression is required for many patients to optimize the release of enzymes from enteric-coated microspheres. Newer high-lipase preparations reduce the number of capsules that patients are required to take on a daily basis [10]. Endocrine insufficiency may respond to oral hypoglycaemic agents in the early stages of the disease but progression to insulin dependency is common in those with severe disease [11].

Pancreatic pain

This is undoubtedly a most difficult problem to treat, often requiring opiate analgesics, sometimes in high dosage. Referral to a pain clinic is often necessary and patients are often best managed by a multidisciplinary approach involving the general practitioner, gastroenterologist, surgeon and an anaesthetist with an interest in pain management. Intractable symptoms should trigger referral to a tertiary centre with a view to assessing the patient for a total pancreatectomy by a dedicated pancreatic surgeon [12].

There is also evidence to suggest that oxygen free radicals play a part in the ongoing damage associated with chronic pancreatitis and that treatment with antioxidants is beneficial.

References

1 Mergener K, Baillie J. Acute pancreatitis. *BMJ* 1998; **316**: 44–8.
2 Ros E, Navarro S, Bru C, Garcia-Puges A, Valderrama R. Occult microlithiasis in 'idiopathic' acute pancreatitis: prevention of relapses by cholecystectomy or ursodeoxycholic acid therapy. *Gastroenterology* 1991; **101**: 1701–9.
3 Wilson C, Imrie CW. Changing patterns of incidence and mortality from acute pancreatitis in Scotland 1961–85. *Br J Surg* 1990; **77**: 731–4.
4 Aggarwal N, Pitchumoni CS, Sivaprasad AV. Evaluating tests for acute pancreatitis. *Am J Gastroenterol* 1990; **85**: 356–61.
5 Neoptolomos JP, Carr-Locke D, London NJ, Bailey IA, James D, Fossard DP. Controlled trial of urgent endoscopic retrograde cholangiopancreatography and endoscopic sphincterotomy versus conservative treatment for acute pancreatitis due to gallstones. *Lancet* 1988; **ii**: 979–83.
6 Welbourne CRB, Beckly DE, Eyre IA. Endoscopic sphincterotomy without cholecystectomy for gallstone pancreatitis. *Gut* 1995; **37**: 119–20.
7 Targarona EM, Ayuso RM, Bordas JM, Ros JM, Pros I, Martinez J, Tetes J, Trias M. Randomised trial of endoscopic sphincterotomy with gallbladder left in situ versus open surgery for common bileduct calculi in high-risk patients. *Lancet* 1996; **347**: 926–9.
8 Wakasugi H, Funakoshi A, Iguchi H. Clinical assessment of pancreatic diabetes caused by chronic pancreatitis. *J Gastroenterol* 1998; **33**: 254–9.
9 Walsh TN, Rode J, Theis BA, Russell RC. Minimal change chronic pancreatitis. *Gut* 1992; **33**: 1566–71.
10 Gan KH, Heijerman HG, Bakker W, Lamers CB. Comparison of a high lipase pancreatic enzyme extract with a regular pancreatin press in adult cystic fibrosis. *Aliment Pharmacol Ther* 1994; **8**: 603–7.
11 von Tirpitz C, Glasbrenner B, Meyer D, Malfertheiner P, Adler G. Comparison of different endocrine stimulation tests in nondiabetic patients with chronic pancreatitis. *Hepatogastroenterology* 1998; **45**: 1111–16.
12 Evans JD, Wilson PG, Carver C *et al*. Outcome of surgery for chronic pancreatitis. *Br J Surg* 1997; **84**: 624–9.

8 Irritable bowel syndrome

Robin Spiller

Key Points

- Irritable bowel syndrome (IBS) affects 15% of the population in a 12-month period.
- The extent of health-care seeking is often predicted by psychological traits.
- Diagnose IBS if frequent abdominal pain and discomfort are present and associated with disturbed bowel habit.
- Investigate if atypical symptoms, new onset at age over 40 or alarm symptoms, e.g. weight loss, rectal bleeding.
- Treatment primarily comprises explanation of the condition.
- Drug treatment has a high placebo effect and should be aimed at the predominant symptom.

Background

It is unlikely that there is a single aetiology underlying the diverse symptoms experienced in irritable bowel syndrome (IBS). We should not therefore expect all patients to show similar features or predisposing factors. A substantial minority develop symptoms acutely in the setting of what appears to be an acute infectious diarrhoea (see below). Specific food intolerances appear to be responsible in a further small subgroup but for the majority the most consistent predisposing factors are psychosocial abnormalities and visceral hypersensitivity, aspects that may well be interrelated.

The effect of mood on gastrointestinal function

Abdominal cramps and diarrhoea as a result of acute anxiety are within the experience of most individuals. Depressed patients have delay in both small bowel and whole gut transit while anxious patients by contrast have an accelerated small bowel transit [1]. Laboratory animals also show accelerated colonic transit when stressed. These effects of mood on symptoms of diarrhoea and abdominal cramps are commonly recognized by patients [2,3]. There is no experimental evidence that IBS patients' colons differ from those of normal subjects in respect to effects of stress. However, altered autonomic reactivity has been noted in IBS, with increased vagal tone being associated with constipation-predominant IBS, while increased sympathetic activity is associated with diarrhoea. Attempts to show distinct altered motility patterns in IBS patients have been unconvincing.

Visceral hypersensitivity

Patients with IBS appear to regard all stimuli coming from their gut in a negative fashion. This is termed negative affective biasing. Over the last 25 years many authors have demonstrated that inflating a balloon in numerous parts of the gut to steadily increasing volumes produces pain in IBS patients at lower threshold volumes than in normal patients. These changes appeared specific to gut stimulation since somatic pain thresholds to cold or electrical cutaneous stimulation are either normal or even increased. However, there does appear to be a degree of anticipation in the responses that subjects report. The bowel does not appear to be inherently sensitive but rather the interpretation of the stimuli appears abnormal.

Recently functional magnetic resonance imaging and positron emission tomography techniques have been developed to measure brain activation from cerebral blood flow. These studies have demonstrated an abnormal pattern of activation in the cortex of IBS patients in response both to balloon distension and to sham distension. While healthy subjects show activation of the anterior cingulate cortex in response to a painful stimulus, IBS patients show a blunted response in this area but significant activation of the left prefrontal cortex. This activation is as great for a sham stimulus as for the real one, indicating that it is the central reaction to the anticipated stimulus that is abnormal. Similar abnormal central processing of visceral stimuli has been reported in other painful functional disorders such as fibromyalgia. This provides a mechanism that could explain the link between psychological states and altered visceral perception in IBS.

Psychological abnormalities

Depending on the setting in which patients are examined there is a higher incidence of anxiety, depression and sleep disturbance. These abnormalities are more striking in a secondary or tertiary referral setting than in general practice. Psychological abnormalities are more common in patients with long-standing symptoms [4].

Several studies have linked the onset of IBS symptoms to a stressful event such as employment difficulties, a family death, a surgical procedure or marital stress [5]. A history of sexual abuse often combined with physical abuse, in both childhood and subsequent adult life, has been reported in 20–30% of patients with IBS seen in a hospital setting [6,7]. Adverse life events prior to the onset of IBS symptoms were also reported significantly more commonly than in patients with organic disease [8]. Another study reported that, although the frequency of adverse events was similar in IBS and patients with organic disease, anxiety provoked by such events preceded the onset of symptoms in two-thirds of IBS patients but only 25% of patients with organic disease.

Post-infective IBS

Some IBS patients report that their symptoms began after an acute gastrointestinal illness, a feature that appears to predict a better prognosis and less psychological abnormalities. Two recent studies have confirmed persistent bowel dysfunction in one-quarter to one-third of patients with documented bacterial dysentery due to *Campylobacter*, *Shigella* and *Salmonella* [9]. The risk factors for persistent symptoms included a more severe and prolonged initial illness as well as higher anxiety.

Diet

Patients often report that certain foods trigger their symptoms and this is confused with food allergy. This can lead to progressively more restricted diets, often aided by complementary practitioners.

Studies that have used dietary restriction followed by sequential introduction of single foods have reported specific food intolerances in between one-third and two-thirds of IBS patients [10,11]. The commonest intolerances reported in the UK involve dairy products (30%) followed by onions, wheat, chocolate and coffee. Malabsorption of osmotically active fermentable carbohydrates such as lactose and fructose are known to cause typical IBS symptoms such as bloating, cramps and diarrhoea. Adult-acquired hypolactasia is common in the UK and the USA with an incidence of 10% in those of northern

European descent, rising to 60% in Asians and 90% in Chinese [12]. Regional variations in dairy intake may account for the varied benefit reported with lactose-free diets. In Denmark, with a traditionally high intake of dairy products, a low lactose diet has been reported to produce improvement in over a half of adults with symptoms of IBS and objective evidence of lactose malabsorption.

Validation of the existence of true food intolerance is very hard to perform since placebo response cannot be excluded unless one performs a double-blind food challenge. When suspected foods are disguised or delivered by nasogastric intubation only a minority of patients can correctly identify foods they believe to trigger their symptoms. It follows that much of the supposed food allergy relates to the patient's belief rather than something that happens locally in the bowel. Recent advances in neuro-immunology have indicated that mast cell degranulation and other immune phenomena can be psychologically triggered so it is possible that patient's beliefs about food can activate an immunological response.

The extent of the problem

Overview

8

Irritable bowel syndrome symptoms are within the experience of most people. Thus two-thirds of Danish females and over half the males admitted to some combination of abdominal pain, altered stool consistency and abdominal distension. However, this figure falls to 20 and 11%, respectively, if the symptoms were required to occur more frequently than once a month. If relief by defecation is included within the definition the prevalence fell to 7% and 5% for women and men, respectively. Thus IBS is akin to having raised blood pressure, something that many people have to a greater or lesser extent and which may need treatment if it exceeds certain limits. It follows therefore that what doctors see is the tip of the iceberg and many of the features of IBS relate to the characteristics of individuals who seek medical help

Epidemiology

The prevalence of IBS in the community depends on the criteria used. Most authors have used the presence of three or more Manning criteria, a diagnostic classification previously commonly used and now superseded by the Rome criteria (Table 8.1). The Rome criteria have

Table 8.1 Criteria for diagnosing IBS.

Rome criteria (revised version) [13]
At least 3 months of recurrent symptoms of abdominal pain or discomfort: • relieved with defecation; or   • associated with a change in stool frequency; or   • associated with a change in stool consistency   **and**   Two or more of the following, at least 25% of occasions or days: • altered stool frequency   • altered stool form   • altered stool passage   • passage of mucus   • bloating or distension

Table 8.2 Frequency of IBS in the USA and the UK using three Manning criteria or the Rome criteria.

Source	Group characteristics	N	Diagnosis	IBS (%) Total	Women	Men
Talley [13]	US white	835	3 Manning	12.8	13.6	12.1
Heaton [14]	UK white, urban	1896	3 Manning	9.5	13.0	5.0
Drossman [16]	US 95% white	5430	Rome	9.4	14.5	7.7

been further revised so that the second set of symptoms are supportive rather than obligatory for the diagnosis [32]. They do require two of the three initial features to be present and are as such more specific but less sensitive.

The overall incidence by this approach is between 9 and 15% [14–17] (Table 8.2).

Presentation and common symptoms

Consultation rates

The cost and incentives for consultation with physicians varies with

8

the health-care system. Studies based in the UK indicate that between one-third and a half of patients [15,18] have consulted their general practitioner. Patients in the USA on average report a total of 5.5 physician visits in the last year of which one-third were for gastrointestinal (GI) symptoms [17]. This same survey found that females were more likely to consult than males, a feature which is seen in most studies throughout the world [19,20].

Several studies have attempted to predict consulting behaviour. Perhaps as would be expected consultation is increased in those with more severe pain, more urgency [15,21] and rectal bleeding [22]. Fewer elderly sufferers with IBS symptoms were found to attend a physician in the USA but why this was so is not clear [23]. Patient factors are not the only determinant, and in the UK consultation rates varied widely from 18 to 38% of patients between different general practitioners [22], so plainly practitioner attitude is also an important variable.

Several studies have indicated that IBS patients also consult more frequently than normal for non-GI disorders (1.5 vs. 0.6 consultations per year) [24]. It seems logical that patients who are anxious are more likely to seek reassurance by consulting a physician but this has not been easy to demonstrate consistently. An Australian study found that, in a system where health care is free, if symptoms are severe the majority (73%) of patients will consult [25]. The best predictor of consultation in this study was the severity of abdominal pain. Under these circumstances neuroticism and pyschological morbidity did not predict attendance. However, whether patients get referred on from their general practitioner may well be influenced by psychological traits. Once they have reached a hospital outpatients, patients with IBS tend to have significantly more anxiety, depression and somatization compared with normals but similar degrees of psychological abnormalities when compared with patients with other organic diseases [26]. This suggests that psychological traits predict health-care seeking but cannot be used to predict the diagnosis.

The transition from primary to secondary care has recently been analysed in some detail in a study from the Netherlands [2]. The authors found that those attending outpatients reported more severe and more frequent abdominal pain. Outpatients were more likely to attribute their complaints to somatic causes, whereas primary care patients were more likely to attribute their complaints to stress and hence probably more likely to accept reassurance from their primary care physician.

Psychological abnormalities appear more prominent in tertiary referral centres in the USA where patients were found to score higher on hypochondriasis, depression and hysteria, and report fewer positive life experiences [27]. Perhaps not surprisingly it appears that the further one moves away from the general practice setting the more psychological problems are detected. Predictably it appears that it is the more anxious patients who are less likely to accept reassurance and seek further referrals including non-gastroenterological ones. This feature may also explain why IBS patients are over-represented in gynaecology clinics [28] and more likely to undergo unnecessary surgical procedures [29].

Clinical diagnosis and investigations

It should be noted that many patients with abdominal pain and disturbed bowel habit do not exactly fit these criteria [30], yet their clinical course is similar. Some have argued that the above criteria are cumbersome and difficult to use. Recently, the simplified Swedish criterion of 'frequent abdominal pain or discomfort associated with disturbed bowel habit' [31] has been shown to correlate well with both, and approximate to the new Rome II criteria [32].

Management

Current guidelines

8

The American Gastroenterological Association has published guidelines [33] and the British Society of Gastroenterology's version will shortly be available for public consultation [34]. Both agree that, in this benign, non-life-threatening condition, education, reassurance and establishing an effective therapeutic relationship between patient and physician are an essential part of management. This begins with a positive diagnosis of IBS based on established criteria and associated key factors. These include frequent consultations for non-GI disorders, a history of more than 2 years and the absence of any sinister features such as weight loss or rectal bleeding. Atypical symptoms or symptoms developing *de novo* in a patient over the age of 40 should indicate the need for further investigations, including a barium enema to exclude carcinoma of the colon. This is particularly important, as it is a potentially fatal condition, the outcome of which depends critically upon the stage at which it is first detected.

Treatment

1 If the clinical scenario is typical then treatment should include an explanation of the symptomatology together with reassurance that IBS does not lead to other serious diseases.

2 Medication directed at the predominant symptom is relatively successful, although much of the success is a non-specific placebo effect.

3 Although widely used, the number of subjects responding specifically to antispasmodics is small.

4 Tricyclic antidepressants are effective particularly for pain, especially when patients are overtly depressed.

5 Constipation can be treated with increased dietary fibre, with or without ispaghula supplements, always bearing in mind the fact that up to 50% of IBS patients find their symptoms are aggravated by bran.

6 Diarrhoeal symptoms can be successfully treated with loperamide 2–4 mg up to four times daily.

7 Psychological treatments are more time consuming and usually only initiated when symptoms are severe or there are associated psychiatric disorders such as major depression. Psychotherapy, cognitive behavioural therapy, hypnosis and relaxation are all effective in reducing abdominal pain and diarrhoea and their benefit appears long lasting.

8 Management requires regular review. Progressive symptoms in spite of treatment would be an indication for further referral.

Management guidelines

1 Patients under the age of 40 with abdominal pain associated with altered stool frequency and consistency are likely to have IBS, particularly if symptoms are long standing (more than 2 years), of fluctuating intensity, and not associated with anorexia, weight loss, anaemia or rectal bleeding.

2 The association with other functional GI symptoms either present or past, together with multiple non-GI symptoms, predicts a high probability of IBS.

3 Treatments should involve reassurance and a simple explanation of visceral hypersensitivity.

4 Reassessment some weeks later should find many patients with symptoms resolving.

5 Those in whom symptoms persist should have psychosocial issues discussed and this may reveal underlying psychopathology which requires treatment.

6 Trials of either tricyclic antidepressants or antispasmodics, lopera-mide or fibre may be appropriate at this stage depending on the predominant symptom.

7 After further review, a form of psychological treatment may be justified if symptoms persist.

8 If there is progression in symptoms, the patient should be referred for further investigations.

9 Patients with age >40 at onset, who have a short history with pro-gressive symptoms, are at increased risk of organic disease and usually require further investigations. This may include full blood count, erythrocyte sedimentation rate, and a thyroid function test performed in the general practice setting with or without a barium enema.

10 If these investigations are negative but symptoms progress then it would be appropriate to refer for sigmoidoscopy, which is probably best performed prior to a barium enema to reliably exclude local causes of bleeding and diarrhoea, including colitis and haemorrhoids.

11 Patients referred to hospital have a higher proportion of organic disease and generally further investigations are indicated including:

   (a) screening for thyroid disorders;

   (b) chronic gastrointestinal infections (e.g. giardiasis); and

   (c) occult inflammatory bowel disease particularly Crohn's disease.

These investigations reveal a low incidence of abnormality, of the order of 1–2% [35], but are important since they reveal treatable conditions and make significant changes in management.

12 Testing for lactose intolerance yields a much higher proportion of abnormal results (25%) but these are only significant in a small propor-tion of patients who drink substantial amounts (>240 ml) of milk daily.

13 When diarrhoea predominates, antiendomysial antibodies can be useful to reduce the risk of missing occult coeliac disease.

14 If stool volumes are increased, a laxative screen may also be appropriate.

15 If symptoms persist and no new diagnosis is uncovered, further reassurance and attention to psychiatric features are indicated as dis-cussed above.

References

1 Gorard DA, Gomborone JE, Libby GW, Farthing MJ. Intestinal transit in anxiety and depression [see comments]. *Gut* 1996; **39**: 551–5.

2 Van Der Horst HE, Van Dulmen AM, Schellevis FG, van Eijk JT, Fennis JF, Bleijenberg G. Do patients with irritable bowel syndrome in primary care really differ from outpatients with irritable bowel syndrome? *Gut* 1997; **41**: 669–74.

3 Whitehead WE, Crowell MD, Robinson JC, Heller BR, Schuster MM. Effects of stressful life events on bowel symptoms: Subjects with irritable bowel syndrome compared with subjects without bowel dysfunction. *Gut* 1992; **33**: 825–30.

4 Lembo T, Fullerton S, Diehl D *et al.* Symptom duration in patients with irritable bowel syndrome. *Am J Gastroenterol* 1996; **91**: 898–905.

5 Corney RH, Stanton R. Physical symptom severity, psychological and social dysfunction in a series of outpatients with irritable bowel syndrome. *J Psychosom Res* 1990; **34**: 483–91.

6 Delvaux M, Denis P, Allemand H. Sexual abuse is more frequently reported by IBS patients than by patients with organic digestive diseases or controls. Results of a multicentre inquiry. *Eur J Gastroenterol Hepatol* 1997; **9**: 345–52.

7 Talley NJ, Boyce PM, Jones M. Is the association between the irritable bowel syndrome and abuse explained by neuroticism? A population based study. *Gut* 1998; **42**: 47–53.

8 Creed F, Craig T, Farmer R. Functional abdominal pain, psychiatric illness, and life events. *Gut* 1988; **29**: 235–42.

9 Neal KR, Hebden JM, Spiller RC. Prevalence of gastrointestinal symptoms six months after bacterial gastroenteritis and risk factors for the development of irritable bowel syndrome: postal survey of patients. *BMJ* 1997; **314**: 779–82.

10 Nanda R, James R, Smith H, Dudley CRK, Jewel DP. Food intolerance and the irritable bowel syndrome. *Gut* 1989; **30**: 1099–104.

11 Jones VA, McLaughlan P, Shorthouse M, Workman E, Hunter JO. Food intolerance: a major factor in the pathogenesis of irritable bowel syndrome. *Lancet* 1982; **ii**: 1115–17.

12 Simoons FJ. The geographic hypothesis and lactose malabsorption a weighing of the evidence. *Dig Dis Sci* 1978; **23**: 963–79.

13 Drossman DA, Thompson WG, Talley NJ, Funch-Jensen P, Janssens J, Whitehead WE. Identification of subgroups of functional gastrointestinal disorders. *Gastroenterol Int* 1990; **3**: 159–72.

14 Talley NJ, Zinsmeister AR, Van Dyke C, Melton LJ III. Epidemiology of colonic symptoms and the irritable bowel syndrome. *Gastroenterology* 1991; **101**: 927–34.

15 Heaton KW, O'Donnell LD, Braddon FM *et al.* Symptoms of irritable bowel syndrome in a British urban community: Consulters and nonconsulters. *Gastroenterology* 1992; **102**: 1962–7.

16 Taub E, Cuevas JL, Cook IIE, Crowell M, Whitehead WE. Irritable bowel syndrome defined by factor analysis. Gender and race comparisons. *Dig Dis Sci* 1995; **40**: 2647–55.

17 Drossman DA, Li Z, Andruzzi E *et al.* U.S. householder survey of functional gastrointestinal disorders. Prevalence, sociodemography, and health impact. *Dig Dis Sci* 1993; **38**: 1569–80.

18 Jones R. Irritable bowel syndrome. *Biomed Pharmacother* 1992; **46**: 426.

19 Jeong H, Lee HR, Yoo BC, Park SM. Manning criteria in irritable bowel syndrome: its diagnostic significance. *Korean J Intern Med* 1993; **8**: 34–9.

20 Kapoor KK, Nigam P, Rastogi CK, Kumar A, Gupta AK. Clinical profile of irritable bowel syndrome. *Indian J Gastroenterol* 1985; **4**: 15–6.

21 Heaton KW, Ghosh S, Braddon FM. How bad are the symptoms and bowel dysfunction of patients with the irritable bowel syndrome? A prospective, controlled study with emphasis on stool form. *Gut* 1991; **32**: 73–9.

22 Jones R, Lydeard S. Irritable bowel syndrome in the general population. *BMJ* 1992; **304**: 87–90.

23 Talley NJ, O'Keefe EA, Zinsmeister AR, Melton LJ III. Prevalence of gastrointestinal symptoms in the elderly: a population-based study. *Gastroenterology* 1992; **102**: 895–901.

24 Sandler RS, Drossman DA, Nathan HP, McKee DC. Symptom complaints and health care seeking behavior in subjects with bowel dysfunction. *Gastroenterology* 1984; **87**: 314–18.

25 Talley NJ, Boyce PM, Jones M. Predictors of health care seeking for irritable bowel syndrome: a population based study [see comments]. *Gut* 1997; **41**: 394–8.

26 Smith RC, Greenbaum DS, Vancouver JB *et al.* Psychosocial factors are associated with health care seeking rather than diagnosis in irritable bowel syndrome. *Gastroenterology* 1990; **98**: 293–301.

27 Drossman DA, McKee DC, Sandler RS *et al.* Psychosocial factors in the irritable bowel syndrome. A multivariate study of patients and nonpatients with irritable bowel syndrome. *Gastroenterology* 1988; **95**: 701–8.

28 Prior A, Wilson K, Whorwell PJ, Faragher EB. Irritable bowel syndrome in the gynecological clinic. Survey of 798 new referrals. *Dig Dis Sci* 1989; **34**: 1820–4.

29 Burns DG. The risk of abdominal surgery in irritable bowel syndrome. *S Afr Med J* 1986; **70**: 91.

30 Thompson WG, Dotevall G, Drossman DA, Heaton KW, Kruis. Irritable bowel syndrome. Guidelines for the diagnosis. *Gastroenterol Int* 1989; **2**: 92–5.

31 Agreus L, Talley NJ, Svardsudd K, Nyren O, Tibblin G, Jones MP. Is it possible to simplify the definition of the irritable bowel syndrome in population based studies and clinical practice? *Gastroenterology* 1998; **114**: A2–A2 (Abstract).

32 Thompson WG, Longstreth GF, Drossman DA, Heaton KW, Irvine EJ, Miller-Lessener SA. Functional bowel disorders and abdominal pain. *Gut* 1999; **45** (511): 143–7.

33 Drossman DA, Whitehead WE, Camilleri M. American gastroenterological association medical position statement: Irritable bowel syndrome. *Gastroenterology* 1997; **112**: 2118–19.

34 Jones J *et al.* British Society of Gastroenterology Guidelines for the management of functional bowel disorders with special reference to irritable bowel syndrome. *Gut* 2000; in press.

35 Hamm LR, Sorrells SC, Harding JP. Utility of screening tests in irritable bowel syndrome. Its value in the exclusion of organic disease. *Gastroenterology* 1998; **112**: A1082.

8

9 Coeliac disease and malabsorption problems

John Silcock

Key Points

- Prevalence is 1 in 300 of the adult population.
- Usual presentation in adults is with iron deficiency anaemia, tiredness or gastrointestinal symptoms.
- Initial diagnosis is by endomysial antibodies, confirmation by intestinal biopsy.
- Mainstay of treatment is a lifelong gluten-free diet.
- Consider screening patients with insulin-dependent diabetes melitus, infertility, Down's syndrome and affected family members.

Background

The classic clinical and histological features of coeliac disease were first described over a century ago by Gee [1]. There have been references to a disorder similar to coeliac disease in ancient Greek medical texts from the time of Hippocrates. It was not, however, until Dicke in 1950 that the association with wheat gluten was recognized [2].

Coeliac disease or gluten-sensitive enteropathy is an inflammatory condition affecting the small bowel. There is an inappropriate, immuno-logically mediated response to protein components found in wheat, barley and rye but not oats [3]. (Oats may become contaminated with wheat flour during manufacture, storage and packaging processes resulting in apparent intolerance.) The inflammatory processes that occur result in the characteristic histological appearance of villous atrophy, crypt hyperplasia and lymphocyte infiltration. The inflammatory changes regress and the morphology returns to normal following the adoption of a gluten-free diet (GFD). The loss of absorptive capacity results in the well-recognized clinical features of malabsorption such as diarrhoea and weight loss and also in the less commonly recognized complications of anaemia (which may be iron and/or folate deficient) and osteopenia (secondary to calcium malabsorption). The chronic inflammatory process is believed to be responsible for the increased incidence of gastrointestinal malignancies and non-Hodgkin's type lymphomas seen in this group.

The extent of the problem

The prevalence of coeliac disease in the UK was estimated previously as between 1 : 1000 and 1 : 1500. A general practitioner may therefore expect to have one or two patients with coeliac disease in his or her list and a typical district general hospital usually cares for about 150 patients. However, this is likely to be an underestimate of the population prevalence because of the difficulties in identifying the potentially much larger group of asymptomatic patients. Serological surveys with follow-up duodenal biopsies in those patients with positive immunological markers have reported the prevalence to be as great as 1 : 150 in Ireland and 1 : 300 in Italy [4,5]. A recent case-finding study in the UK using endomysial antibodies also reported a prevalence of 1 in 300 in the screened population [6]. The criteria for screening included anaemia, irritable bowel syndrome, autoimmune disorders and fatigue.

Presentation and common symptoms

9

Coeliac disease is a *common* condition and responds readily to a simple dietary restriction. If undetected, it is potentially a cause of significant morbidity and indeed mortality.

Such a statement, at first glance, would appear to be contrary to the personal experience of most practitioners. The classic presentation of a child or young adult with a history of weight loss, diarrhoea and perhaps growth or developmental retardation, although well described in undergraduate texts, is not common. In adults coeliac disease should be considered in those who are tired and those who have iron deficiency anaemia, as well as those with gastrointestinal symptoms. One in five patients joining the Coeliac Society is over 60 years of age and in these patients anaemia is the commonest presenting symptom [7]. There appears to be a much larger group of patients with subclinical coeliac disease who are at risk of complications. This has given rise to the concept of a coeliac disease 'iceberg' with only those patients with gastrointestinal symptoms floating above the water level of clinical detection.

Clinical diagnosis and investigations

The optimal investigation for establishing the initial diagnosis is the endomysial antibody test, performed on a venous sample. Those who prove positive should then be offered endoscopy and duodenal biopsy. This has replaced the Crosby Capsule as a means of obtaining tissue for microscopy. A characteristic morphology of the duodenal folds in patients with untreated coeliac disease has been described and keenly observant endoscopists may describe scalloped edges to the duodenal folds.

Conditions associated with coeliac disease

Dermatitis herpetiformis

Dermatitis herpetiformis is a blistering skin disorder affecting the extensor surfaces. Its association with coeliac disease is well recognized. IgA deposition within the dermis of unaffected skin is characteristic. Small bowel villous atrophy with crypt hyperplasia is observed in 75% of patients with dermatitis herpetiformis and minor mucosal changes are often observed in the remainder [8]. The treatment of this condition is the adoption of a GFD and additionally dapsone or sulphapyridine may be required. The skin condition tends to improve over a period of 2 years following which the dapsone may be discontinued and it tends to remain in remission while strict adherence to the GFD is maintained.

9

Insulin-dependent diabetes mellitus

There is no increase in frequency of coeliac disease in patients with non-insulin-dependent diabetes mellitus (NIDDM) [9]. The prevalence of coeliac disease on screening of patients with insulin-dependent diabetes mellitus (IDDM), however, is greatly increased and in studies varies between 1.0 and 7.8% [10,11]. Iron deficiency is the most common biochemical abnormality and glucose control is not usually adversely affected. Adherence to a GFD may prove problematical as the standard dietary regimens for IDDM are typically high in gluten.

Down's syndrome

Coeliac disease, as confirmed by duodenal biopsies following initial serological screening, is common in Down's syndrome patients and in one series the prevalence was as high as 9% [12]. There is also an association between coeliac disease and epilepsy, learning disorders and cerebral calcification.

Coeliac disease may also present as a manifestation of deficiency states.

Metabolic bone disease

Patients may present with osteoporosis (secondary to calcium malabsorption) and less commonly osteomalacia (secondary to vitamin D malabsorption) often in the absence of significant gastrointestinal symptoms [13]. Osteoporosis in men or premenopausal women should be taken as an indication for screening but advanced age does not exclude the diagnosis. Even in those patients not presenting with metabolic bone disease, bone mineral density has been demonstrated to be significantly lower in patients at presentation than in age- and sex-matched controls. Following introduction of a GFD, there is a significant increase in bone mineral density over the first 12 months, although this still remains suboptimal [14]. Dietary supplements during this period would be advisable.

Anaemia

Anaemia secondary to iron or folate deficiency is another common route of presentation. The mechanism is partly one of malabsorption and also increased losses due to increased enterocyte turnover. Folate deficiency may be exacerbated by associated anorexia and decreased intake.

Complications of coeliac disease

The complications of untreated coeliac disease are usually long term (Table 9.1). They may be secondary to the ensuing deficiencies in iron, folate and calcium absorption, namely anaemia and osteoporosis and the associated increased risk of fractures. Malabsorption can result in symptoms of altered bowel habit, abdominal pain and weight loss. Other less commonly recognized complications include subfertility. This may result in reversible infertility in men and infertility and increased risk of spontaneous abortions in women. A study of female patients

Table 9.1 Complications of coeliac disease.

- Osteoporosis
- Anaemia
- Infertility
- Malignancies—non-Hodgkin's lymphoma, small bowel adenocarcinoma

with unexplained infertility found a prevalence of coeliac disease of 4.1% [15]. This was 10 times the prevalence expected.

Malignancy

Overall, there is a twofold increase in the risk of malignancy in patients with coeliac disease. Commonly, the malignancy is a lymphoma (usually a non-Hodgkin's type) but cancers of the mouth, pharynx and oesophagus is recognized as is adenocarcinoma of the small bowel, an otherwise rare tumour. Patients who have adhered to a strict GFD for 5 or more years reduce their risk to that of the non-coeliac population [16]. Therefore, it is recommended that the diet should be life long and strictly adhered to.

Follow-up and prognosis

Follow-up in hospital has formed part of the traditional management of coeliac patients. It is usual practice to repeat the duodenal biopsies 6 months following commencement of the GFD to confirm resolution of the morphological changes and also to repeat endoscopy and duodenal biopsies at times of symptom relapse.

Steroids have been used in addition to GFD previously but are not widely prescribed now. Once established on a GFD, dietary supplements of iron, calcium or folate should no longer be necessary although these are often prescribed at the time of diagnosis to correct specific deficiency states. It has now been established that the increased risk of malignancy falls to background levels after 5 years. Therefore, the argument could be made for further follow-up to continue in the general practice setting with referral back for assessment should problems arise despite apparent adherence to the GFD. It is likely that, as a result of increased awareness of the asymptomatic 'latent' coeliac, more cases are diagnosed and that a shift of care in the primary-care setting will occur.

9

Screening and prevention

The basis of screening

Coeliac disease is an immunologically mediated inflammatory process and circulating antibodies have formed the basis of screening.

Antigliadin antibodies are often used for initial screening. Gluten is the protein extract of wheat flour and gliaden is that component of gluten that is soluble in 70% alcohol. IgA and IgG antibody titres are usually measured. Typically there is a high titre of antigliadin IgA present often in association with a raised IgG titre. IgA deficiency occurs in 1 in 50 patients with coeliac disease giving rise to a solitary raised IgG in these patients [17]. Antigliadin antibodies in high titres are present in less than 5% of non-coeliacs but in 80% of untreated adult and 95% of untreated child coeliacs. As a screening method they are relatively cheap and widely available.

Antiendomysial antibodies are principally directed against tissue transglutaminases. Endomysial antibodies are more sensitive and specific than antigliadin antibodies and form the second tier of many screening strategies. Positive antiendomysial antibodies are found in less than 1% of non-coeliacs and in 95% of untreated coeliacs of all ages. Some laboratories are now offering endomysial antibody assays on their own.

Who should be screened?

In a condition that presents classically in only a minority of cases, a knowledge of hereditary factors and associated conditions is necessary to target the screening strategy to the at-risk population.

Coeliac disease is associated with HLA class II haplotypes *DR3-DQ2* and *DR5/7-DQ2*. These genes code for cell-surface molecules which bind and present antigenic peptides to T cells and are associated with autoimmune disorders (such as IDDM and autoimmune thyroid disease). Whilst specific gene markers are not widely available, 10% of first-degree relatives will also have coeliac disease and can be screened. If positive endomysial antibodies are found, referral for endoscopy and duodenal biopsies should be made.

Useful resources

Guidelines of the British Society of Gastroenterology:
  http://www.bsg.org.uk/clinical/data/gmpcd.htm
  Coeliac Society: http://www.coeliac.co.uk/
Sites with useful patient information, links and recipes:
  http://www.celiac.com/
  http://www.panix.com/~donwiss/
  http://www.niddk.nih.gov/health/digest/pubs/celiac/index.htm

References

1 Gee S. On the coeliac disease. *St Bart Hosp Rep* 1888; **24**: 17–20.
2 Dicke WK. Coeliake. MD Thesis, Utrecht 1950.
3 Srinivasan U, Leonard N, Jones E, Kasarda DD, Weir DG, O'Farrelly C, Feighery C. Absence of oats toxicity in adult coeliac disease. *BMJ* 1996; **313**: 1300–1.
4 Johnston SD, Watson RG, McMillan SA, McMaster D, Evans A. Preliminary results from follow up of a large-scale population survey of antibodies to gliadin, reticulin and endomysium. *Acta Paediatr Suppl* 1996; **412**: 61–4.
5 Catassi C, Ratsch IM, Fabiani E *et al.* Coeliac disease in the year 2000: exploring the iceberg. *Lancet* 1994; **343**: 200–3.
6 Hin H, Bird G, Fisher P, Mahy N, Jewell D. Coeliac disease in primary care. a case finding study. *BMJ* 1999; **318**: 164–7.
7 Hankey GL, Holmes GK. Coeliac disease in the elderly. *Gut* 1994; **35**: 65–7.
8 Reunala T, Kosnai I, Karpati S. Dermatitis herpetiformis: jejunal findings and skin response to gluten-free diet. *Arch Dis Child* 1984; **59**: 517–22.
9 Page SR *et al.* The prevalence of coeliac disease in adult diabetes mellitus. *Q J Med* 1994; **87**: 631–7.
10 Koletzko S *et al.* Prevalence of coeliac disease in diabetic children and adolescents. a multicentre study. *Eur J Pediatr* 1988; **148**: 113–17.
11 De Vitis I *et al.* Coeliac disease (CD) and insulin dependent diabetes mellitus (IDDM). A multicentre study. *Gastroenterology* 1996; **110**: A13.
12 Papadatou *et al.* Endomysial and antigliadin antibodies in patients with Down's syndrome. *Dev Brain Dysfunction* 1996; **9**: 129–32.
13 Shaker JL, Brickner RC, Findling JW *et al.* Hypocalcaemia and skeletal disease as presenting features of coeliac disease. *Arch Intern Med* 1997; **157**: 1013–16.
14 McFarlane XA, Bhalla AK, Robertson DA. Effect of a gluten-free diet on osteopenia in adults with newly diagnosed coeliac disease. *Gut* 1996; **39**: 180–4.
15 Collin P, Vilska S, Heinonen PK. Infertility and coeliac disease. *Gut* 1996; **39**: 382–4.
16 Holmes GK *et al.* Malignancy in coeliac disease—effect of a gluten free diet. *Gut* 1989; **30**: 333–8.
17 Dickey W, McMillan SA, McCrum EE, Evans AE. Association between serum levels of total IgA and IgA class endomysial and antigliadin antibodies: implications for coeliac disease screening. *Eur J Gastroenterol Hepatol* 1997; **9**: 559–62.

9

10 Inflammatory bowel disease

John Mansfield

Key Points

- Prevalence is 200 per 100 000 in the UK.
- Classic symptoms are diarrhoea, abdominal pain and rectal bleeding.
- Initial presentation may be indistinguishable from irritable bowel syndrome.
- Initial investigations comprise stool culture, full blood count and sigmoidoscopy.

Background

Ulcerative colitis and Crohn's disease remain disorders of unknown aetiology despite much research. There have been many hypotheses including specific infections, environmental agents or genetically dysregulated mucosal immunity, but none has yet been convincingly proven. Animal models exist but have not shed much light on the cause of the human disease.

Manipulation of mouse genes has provided some intriguing clues in quite unexpected directions. These experiments have demonstrated that in mice, disruption of single genes controlling cytokines, such as interleukin 10, can produce severe gut-specific inflammation, which is dependent on the presence of normal laboratory bacteria [1]. More recently, manipulation of transgenic mice to specifically damage the cells of the enteric nervous system has been shown to produce a patchy jejunoileitis, suggesting that the enteric nervous system may be a key component of normal mucosal integrity [2]. At present these mouse models of inflammatory bowel disease (IBD) cannot be interpreted as more than signposts for further investigations into the aetiology of the human diseases.

The extent of the problem

Epidemiology and prevalence of inflammatory bowel disease

The incidence of ulcerative colitis and Crohn's disease varies between populations, being high in Scandinavia, the UK, North America, Australia and much of north-west Europe. Areas of demonstrably low incidence appear to be Japan, Israel, Spain and Italy. Within Europe the incidence of both ulcerative colitis and Crohn's disease varies by at least fivefold. The incidence of ulcerative colitis in most populations is roughly double that for Crohn's disease. Incidence rates for both diseases are maximal at the beginning of the third decade of life [3].

The prevalence of inflammatory bowel disease in the UK is around 200 per 100 000 population, some studies reporting higher rates [16]. This suggests that very few practices will have no cases and, even in areas with high prevalence, more than a handful on any general practitioner's list would be unusual.

Inflammatory bowel disease and smoking

There have been few hard clues as to the cause of IBD from descriptive studies of the epidemiology. Smoking habit, however, has a consistent association, ulcerative colitis being associated with non-smoking and Crohn's disease with smoking. The magnitude of these effects is about equal, smoking doubling the risk of Crohn's disease and halving that of ulcerative colitis. Furthermore, the recurrence of Crohn's disease after surgery is also strongly associated with continued smoking, so successful persuasion to give up smoking may be of more value than much prescribed medical therapy [4].

Inflammatory bowel disease and oral contraception

Apart from smoking, the only consistent epidemiological factor of importance to these diseases is the weak association of both Crohn's disease and ulcerative colitis with the use of oral contraceptives. Several studies have found about a 50% increase in the risk of IBD with oral contraceptive use, but it remains unclear whether this is a directly causal relationship, or the effect of a confounding factor [5]. There is little evidence to suggest that oral contraceptives should be stopped or avoided in women with either Crohn's disease or ulcerative colitis,

10

Table 10.1 Extent of disease in Crohn's disease and ulcerative colitis.

Ulcerative colitis

Proctitis	45.2%
Left-sided colitis	33.8%
Total colitis	21.0%

Crohn's disease (more than one site may be involved)

Large bowel	57.5%
Small bowel	26.0%
Ileal	49.0%
Rectal	31.5%

although a recent report has associated their use with an increased risk of relapse in Crohn's disease [6].

Presentation and common symptoms

The range of health problems associated with IBD is wide. The particular problems encountered by any individual are determined by the type and severity of the disease, as well as by the patient's age, activity and aspirations. The symptoms of the diseases themselves—diarrhoea, abdominal pain and rectal bleeding—often have added to them such problems as failure to thrive in children, faecal incontinence and debilitating urgency related to active disease and, in the long term, the increase in the risk of colonic cancer and the anxiety that this can cause. In particular, patients worry about the possibility of needing a per-manent stoma after surgery.

The diseases themselves also span a broad spectrum from trivial proctitis, through total ulcerative colitis, to Crohn's disease affecting any site in the gut (Table 10.1) The diseases are chronic and incurable and each patient therefore requires individual attention and a consistent long-term approach. The potential to improve patients' well-being, by understanding their problems and anxieties, is enormous.

Clinical diagnosis and investigations

Delay to diagnosis

A critical step in the management of these diseases is establishing the correct diagnosis. The average time from onset of symptoms to diagnosis of Crohn's disease is many months to a few years, since mild symptoms of early disease can be indistinguishable from irritable bowel syndrome. Often it is only later, when new features have developed, that the diagnosis can be confirmed.

The delay in final diagnosis can pose problems for the doctor–patient relationship, and unless the problems of diagnosis are understood by the patient it can cause mistrust. Equally, there are inevitably some patients who change diagnoses between Crohn's disease (particularly Crohn's colitis) and ulcerative colitis. It may in some cases be better to keep a generic label of IBD rather than to give the patient the insecurity of a changing diagnosis.

Diagnostic pitfalls

Definite confirmation of a flare-up is essential when a relapse is suspected in a patient known to have IBD. Treatment of infective diarrhoea or post-inflammatory irritable bowel with inappropriate courses of steroids will be likely to do more harm than good. Clinical and laboratory confirmations of disease exacerbations are usually required. These include negative stool cultures, full blood count and sigmoidoscopic examination of the rectal mucosa in the case of colitis. The full blood count will often show a raised platelet count in active disease and possibly also anaemia. The most clinically useful are raised platelets, raised C-reactive protein and raised mucoproteins (A1-acid-glycoprotein) but imaging may be required.

The other serious diagnostic pitfall relates to the increased risk of colon cancer in the colitic colon. This risk is increased in both ulcerative colitis and Crohn's disease and is known to be related to disease extent (defined histologically) and disease duration [7]. The only other factors known to increase the colon cancer risks are IBD-associated sclerosing cholangitis [8] and a family history of colon cancer [9]. The occurrence of a tumour in a colitic bowel will often be mistaken for a flare-up of the initial disease. Thorough investigation, usually by colonoscopy, of any flare-up in long-standing disease is therefore essential.

Screening

The role of colonoscopic screening and surveillance in colitis to detect pre-cancerous dysplasia is controversial. A systematic prospective surveillance programme was found to be unsuccessful in detecting or preventing the development of ulcerative colitis-related tumours [10]. The role of a single screening colonoscopy at 8–10 years after the onset of disease is less controversial than repeated colonoscopic surveillance. A single screening colonoscopy at this time can define disease extent and histological activity, thus identifying patients at highest risk in the future, and can search for the presence of dysplastic mucosa.

Future improvements in molecular pre-malignant markers offer some hope that screening and surveillance can be improved for patients now being diagnosed as new cases of IBD. Understandably, patients may be apprehensive of the increased colon cancer risk and frustrated by the inability of colonoscopic surveillance to prevent it.

Management

The problems posed by IBD are quite diverse and the solutions to them require an individual approach with sympathy and compassion because of the embarrassing nature of many symptoms. The provision of patient information, the establishment of a firm diagnosis, appropriate management of acute attacks and optimal management of remission are all key aspects to management of these disorders [11].

Published guidelines and sources of information

The diversity of IBD and the relatively low prevalence of these diseases have combined to deter writers of guidelines. The British Society of Gastroenterology has published guidelines regarding the histological diagnosis of IBD, but these relate more to problems encountered by gastrointestinal pathologists rather than general practitioners.

10

National Association for Colitis and Crohn's Disease

A key component of the management of any patient with IBD is provision of appropriate information. This should lessen the fear of the unknown future course of their disease, and alleviate the feeling that this is an affliction unique to that individual patient. The patient association NACC (National Association for Colitis and Crohn's Disease) provides invaluable support to many patients. For a modest annual subscription members receive up-to-date leaflets, national and local newsletters and, if they wish, the opportunity to attend meetings and events organized by the local group. A 'can't wait' card is also available which can help with access to toilets in shops, etc., thus relieving some of the anxiety caused by urgency of defecation. The organization also has information leaflets to help with specific circumstances such as helping teachers of pupils with IBD understand the problems that they may encounter.

Treatment

Ulcerative colitis

Less severe cases of ulcerative colitis need careful assessment of severity, followed by treatment with oral steroids or, if the disease is milder, initial treatment with 5-aminosalicylic acid (5ASA) drugs. There are few hard data on which to base an evidence-based discussion as to when oral prednisolone rather than 5ASA is required. Patients who are still at work, or have little disturbance to their pattern of daily activities, can be safely started on 5ASA with escalation to steroids reserved for those who do not improve in the initial few weeks.

Crohn's disease

In Crohn's disease, whether colonic or terminal ileal, steroids are the main agent for treatment of active disease. In contrast to ulcerative colitis the inflammation is typically deeper, often involving the full thickness of the gut wall. Consistent with this, topically liberated 5ASA preparations are of much less value than in ulcerative colitis. Patients who are aware of side effects from prednisolone can be treated with a controlled, ideal-release formulation of budesonide instead, with a reduction in side effects [12].

10

Problems with prednisolone

Side effects from even short courses of prednisolone are considerable [12]. Dose-ranging studies have indicated that 40 mg prednisolone is probably the optimal initial dose [13], reducing over the subsequent 8–12 weeks, depending on clinical response. There is little evidence as to when to start 5ASA drugs if the initial treatment is with steroids, but 5ASA drugs have a definite role in the maintenance of remission of ulcerative colitis, and should be started well before steroids are withdrawn.

In Crohn's disease, osteoporosis is recognized as a complication of the untreated disease, as well as of steroid treatment. Patients who can be identified as at risk of osteoporosis should be considered for hormone replacement therapy (if postmenopausal women), or calcium supplementation with vitamin D. The role of bisphosphonates in these patients is currently under investigation.

Long-term management

Maintenance treatment in Crohn's disease (colonic or small bowel) remains controversial. The benefit from 5ASA drugs appears to be small, with about 16 patients needing to be treated to prevent one relapse. Low-dose steroids for maintenance are not proven to be effective and are probably harmful. Many patients can be followed up with their Crohn's disease in remission on no treatment.

Some small studies have suggested that maintenance treatment with sulfasalazine or mesalazine may reduce the risks of colon cancer in IBD, consistent with the reduced risk of sporadic colorectal tumours associated with aspirin usage [14]. Most patients are on these drugs to reduce the risk of relapse in ulcerative colitis in any case, but this may be a further reason to encourage patients who have been asymptomatic for many years to continue their medical therapy.

Second-line treatment of IBD with immunomodulating drugs such as azathioprine or 6-mercaptopurine should be reserved for patients with persistently active disease in whom surgery is a less desirable option. These patients need close monitoring by both the general practice and the gastroenterologist, and require rapid reassessment if they deteriorate.

The use of rectal preparations in colitis can produce a major improvement in symptom control. The patient should be encouraged to experiment with liquid enemas, foam enemas (aerosol or syringe delivery) or suppositories to define the preparation that suits them best. Both steroid and 5ASA local preparations are now available and are usually equally effective.

Patients often require a constipating agent to give them extra confidence to go out. Either codeine phosphate or loperamide may do this effectively and can be liberating for a patient house-bound by urgency and fear of incontinence. In general, however, constipating agents should be avoided as a regular treatment, as their use will do nothing to improve active inflammation.

Management in childhood

The management of Crohn's disease in childhood presents special problems relating to growth, and should therefore be referred to a

10

suitably interested paediatrician. Within such a speciality setting there is a role for primary treatment of active Crohn's disease with enteral feeding. This can be effective when steroids have failed, or useful when it is desirable to avoid steroids.

Referral

The selection of which patients to refer to hospital clearly depends on the availability of local factors and experience. If colonoscopy and barium radiology are available on an open access basis or performed in the primary-care setting, then patients can be investigated without attending hospital clinics, otherwise referral to gastroenterologists (physicians or surgeons) is advisable.

The management of acute disease depends on the assessment of disease activity. This may be quite different to disease extent. Severity is a function of the degree of systemic upset caused by the inflamed bowel and is classically defined using the criteria of Truelove and Witts [15]. Their definition of severe disease relies on stool frequency, abdominal tenderness, tachycardia and pyrexia. The most severe cases require immediate admission to hospital for intravenous steroids and observation to ensure that, if needed, a colectomy can be performed before life-threatening complications, such as perforation of toxic megacolon, occur. Once admitted such patients should be under joint medical and surgical supervision.

National Association for Colitis and Crohn's Disease

10

Membership of NACC is by contacting the national office at NACC, 4 Beaumont House, Sutton Road, St Albans, Herts, AL1 5HH.
Information and answerphone, 01727 844 296
Fax: 01727 682 550
E-mail: nacc@nacc.org.uk
Website: http://www.nacc.org.uk
Registered charity no: 282732.

References

1 Elson CO, Sartor RB, Tennyson GS, Riddell RH. Experimental models of inflammatory bowel disease. *Gastroenterology* 1995; **109**: 1344–67.
2 Bush TE, Savidge TC, Freeman TC *et al.* Fulminant jejuno-ileitis following ablation of enteric glia in adult transgenic mice. *Cell* 1998; **93**: 189–201.

3 Ekbom A, Helmick C, Zack M, Adami HO. The epidemiology of inflammatory bowel disease: a large population-based study in Sweden. *Gastroenterology* 1991; **100**: 350–8.

4 Sutherland LR, Ramcharan S, Bryant H, Fick G. Effect of cigarette smoking on recurrence of Crohn's disease. *Gastroenterology* 1990; **98**: 1123–8.

5 Godet PG, May GR, Sutherland LR. A meta-analysis of the role of oral contraceptive agents on inflammatory bowel disease. *Gut* 1995; **37**: 668–73.

6 Timmer A, Sutherland LR, Martin F. Oral contraceptive use and smoking are risk factors for relapse in Crohn's disease. The Canadian Mesalazine for Remissions of Crohn's Disease Study Group. *Gastroenterology* 1998; **114**: 1143–50.

7 Ekbom A, Helmick C, Zack M, Adami HO. Ulcerative colitis and colorectal cancer. A population based study. *N Engl J Med* 1990; **323**: 1228–33.

8 Brentnall TA, Hoggitt RC, Rabinovitch PS *et al.* Risk and natural history of colonic neoplasia in patients with primary sclerosing cholangitis and ulcerative colitis. *Gastroenterology* 1996; **110**: 331–8.

9 Nuako KW, Alquist DA, Mahoney DW, Schaid DJ, Siems DM, Lindor NM. Familial predisposition for colorectal cancer in chronic ulcerative colitis: A case control study. *Gastroenterology* 1998; **115**: 1079–83.

10 Lynch DA, Lobo AJ, Sobala GM, Dixon MF, Axon AT. Failure of colonoscopic surveillance in ulcerative colitis. *Gut* 1993; **34**: 1075–80.

11 Mansfield JC, Tanner AR, Bramble MG. Information for patients about inflammatory bowel disease. *J R Coll Physicians Lond* 1997; **31**: 184–7.

12 Campieri M, Ferguson A, Doe W, Persson T, Nilsson L-G. and the Global Budesonide Study Group. Oral budesonide is as effective as oral prednisolone in active Crohn's disease. *Gut* 1997; **41**: 209–14.

13 Baron JH, Connell AM, Kanaghinis TG, Lennard-Jones JE, Avery Jones F. Out-patient treatment of ulcerative colitis. Comparison between three doses of oral prednisone. *BMJ* 1962; **ii**: 441–3.

14 Pinczowski D, Ekbom A, Baron J, Yuen J, Adami H-O. Risk factors for colorectal cancer in patients with ulcerative colitis: a case control study. *Gastroenterology* 1994; **107**: 117–20.

15 Truelove SC, Witts LJ. Cortisone in ulcerative colitis in final report on a therapeutic trial. *BMJ* 1955; **ii**: 1041–8.

16 Rubin GP, Hungin APS, Kelly P, Ling J. Epidemiological features of inflammatory bowel disease in the North of England. *Gastroenterology* 1996; **110** (suppl): 1793.

10

11 Constipation, diarrhoea and minor anal disorders

Greg Rubin

Key Points

- Constipation is common, affecting up to 10% of adults.
- Treatment is aimed at emptying the rectum and then developing a regular bowel habit.
- There is little evidence to support the use of one laxative preparation over another.
- A minority of patients have prolonged gut transit times and are resistant to laxative therapy.

Constipation in children and adults

Constipation is a condition in which bowel evacuations occur infrequently or the faeces are hard and small, or where passage of faeces causes difficulty or pain. The frequency of bowel evacuation varies considerably from person to person and the normal cannot be precisely defined [1]. Encopresis is defined as involuntary bowel movements, in inappropriate places, at a frequency of at least once a month for at least 3 months, for children aged 4 years and older [2].

Prevalence

Constipation with or without encopresis is common in children. It accounts for 3% of consultations to a paediatric outpatient clinic and 25% of paediatric gastroenterology consultations [3]. Among British adults, 10% strain at stool at least 25% of the time and 1% pass fewer than two stools per week.

Features of childhood constipation [1]

• Peak incidence at age 2–4.
• Child's personality—strong-willed, stubborn.
• Parent's personality—overanxious, obsessional or unrealistic standards of hygiene for the child's age.
• Faulty bowel training—ineffective and disorganized, or premature.
• Negativism—other manifestations may include refusal to eat or to sleep.
• Fear—of pain on defecation, possibly with a history of previous anal fissure.
• Organic causes for constipation, such as anatomical, neurological, endocrine and metabolic conditions, are rare.
• Hirschsprung's disease, cystic fibrosis and other forms of malabsorption are the most common organic causes.

Features of adult constipation

• More common in women and the elderly.
• Functional constipation is by far the commonest cause:
  inadequate fibre intake;
  pregnancy;
  old age;
  idiopathic slow transit.
• Drug side effects.
• Rarer causes include structural abnormalities, neurological, endocrine or metabolic disorders, and depression.

Diagnosis

Abdominal distension and faecal masses may be evident on palpation of the abdomen. Digital examination of the rectum is an important part of the assessment and will often reveal a large faecal mass in the rectum. Radiological studies are not routinely indicated in the evaluation of constipation in children [4]. Whole gut transit time is useful in adults, although half of those referred to hospital because of constipation have a normal transit time.

Outcome measures

The following measures, relevant to clinical management, have been used to define successful treatment in children:

11

- defecation three times or more per week;
- soiling less than twice a month;
- no laxatives for at least 4 weeks.

In adults the main outcomes are number of bowel movements per week, stool consistency and abdominal pain.

Intervention options

In children the treatment strategy is threefold, aimed at the removal of faecal impaction, prevention of reaccumulation and reconditioning to normal bowel habits. Counselling and explanation for both child and parents, and behaviour modification, are important adjuncts to medical treatment.

Conventional treatment usually comprises initial rectal washouts with phosphate enemas or bisacodyl suppositories, followed by prolonged treatment with stimulant and lubricant laxatives. However, there are no placebo-controlled trials of the effectiveness of stimulant laxatives in children, although osmotic laxatives have been shown to significantly increase stool frequency [5]. There is no direct evidence of benefit from increasing dietary fibre [6]. Biofeedback training has no effect over and above conventional treatment on the long-term clinical outcome for childhood constipation [7,8].

Most of the placebo-controlled trials of laxatives in adults are small and show only a no-significant trend in favour of treatment. There have been few direct comparisons between different classes of laxatives [9] (Table 11.1).

The initial goal is to empty the rectum and then to develop a regular bowel habit using regular and continuous laxatives to keep the stool

Table 11.1 Laxative groups.

Bulking agents Bran, ispaghula husk
Faecal softeners Paraffin, docusate
Osmotic laxatives Glycerol, lactulose, polyethylene glycol
Stimulant laxatives Senna, bisacodyl, danthron, sodium picosulphate

11

soft. The first step in long-term management is dietary improvement, followed by the cheapest laxative treatment. There is no evidence that danthron laxatives are more effective than other preparations and they should not be routinely used in the treatment of constipation.

Slow transit constipation is usually resistant to these measures. Seen mainly in women and with intervals of a week or more between bowel actions, it is resistant to dietary measures and most patients make intermittent use of stimulant laxatives. Intractable constipation may require surgery. Total colectomy with ileorectal anastomosis will restore normal bowel function to 50% of these patients, but a minority, often those with psychiatric disturbances, will continue to complain of constipation.

Prognosis

Constipation in children can be difficult to treat successfully, requiring prolonged support, explanation and medical treatment. In long-term follow-up studies of children presenting under age 5, 60–70% of children recover; the remainder require laxatives for daily bowel movements or continue soiling for many years [3]. It is not known how many continue to have problems into adult life, although adults presenting with megarectum or megacolon often have a history of bowel problems from childhood.

Diarrhoea

Diarrhoea is a complex entity with multiple causes. One recent classification listed 66 causes in addition to infections. This section will deal only with the initial, largely symptomatic management of acute diarrhoeal illnesses. Diarrhoea can be defined simply as a decrease in consistency or increase in liquidity of the stool. Acute diarrhoea is one of the commonest problems seen in general practice and is usually a brief illness lasting less than 5 days, though it may persist for up to 3 weeks.

Most cases are due to toxin-related food poisoning, viral or bacterial gastroenteritis or dietary indiscretion. Those at high risk of infectious diarrhoea include travellers to developing countries, consumers of shellfish, those indulging in high-risk sexual activity and institutionalized patients.

The mainstay in treatment of acute diarrhoea, whether in children or adults, is replacement of fluid and electrolytes. This can be achieved in infants, young children and the elderly by the use of glucose–electrolyte preparations.

11

Older children and adults should increase their intake of fluids, particularly fruit juice and soups. Fasting is unnecessary. Antidiarrhoeal agents are of limited value but can reduce stool frequency. They should be avoided in children because of their potential for central nervous system side effects and because their use may be a distraction when oral rehydration therapy is the key to effective treatment.

Traveller's diarrhoea

Between 30 and 50% of travellers to developing countries experience traveller's diarrhoea [10]. The most common causes include enterotoxigenic *Escherichia coli*, *Shigella* and *Campylobacter*. The clinical features include three or more unformed stools in a day, accompanied by fever, abdominal cramps or vomiting. Dysentery is defined as these symptoms but with bloody diarrhoea. Traveller's diarrhoea lasts a mean of 4 days although 1–2% last a month or more. Treatment options are shown in Table 11.2.

Table 11.2 Traveller's diarrhoea: treatment options.

Therapy	Effect
Restoration of fluid/electrolyte balance (oral glucose and electrolyte solutions)	Reduce morbidity and mortality, but not duration
Antimicrobial drugs (doxycycline, 4-fluoroquinolones)	Reduce average duration from 4.5 days to 1.5 days
Antidiarrhoeal agents	Reduce stool frequency but not duration

11

Minor anal conditions

Minor anal conditions are common in the community (Table 11.3). It is probable that they are the cause of a significant proportion of the rectal bleeding reported in community prevalence studies, where annual rates in the order of 15% are described. The consultation rate in general practice for piles and anal disorders is 15/1000/year.

95

Table 11.3 Minor anal conditions.

Haemorrhoids
Anal fissure
Fistula *in ano*
Perianal warts
Pruritus ani
Proctalgia fugax

Haemorrhoids and fissures

Haemorrhoids are caused principally by constipation and straining, although their onset in women may be associated with pregnancy. Fissure is most commonly seen in younger patients. It is often associated with anal sphincter spasm but may also occur as a result of local trauma as may be caused by anal intercourse. Curiously, there is a strong association between failure to eat breakfast and haemorrhoids or anal fissure [11]!

The cardinal symptom of haemorrhoids is fresh rectal bleeding which may be copious and occur at the end of defecation. Prolapse and discomfort caused by engorgement can also occur. Anal fissures are the commonest cause of pain, often searing in nature, on defecation. This can be accompanied by slight fresh rectal bleeding, commonly noted on the toilet paper.

Most haemorrhoids respond to an increase in dietary fibre and prevention of constipation and straining [12]. Of the treatment modalities available, rubber band ligation is the recommended initial treatment for all grades of haemorrhoids except those that are permanently prolapsed. Although haemorrhoidectomy shows a better response, it is associated with more complications and pain and should be reserved for those who fail to respond to rubber band ligation. Manual dilatation of the anus, sclerotherapy and infrared coagulation all performed less well in a recent meta-analysis [13].

Anal fissure will often respond to stool softeners and analgesics. Nitroglycerin ointment is effective in decreasing anal sphincter tone and results in healing in 50% of cases [14]. However, it is not available in a commercial preparation in community pharmacies at present. Chronic fissure not responding to these measures is treated surgically by lateral anal sphincterotomy.

11

Fistula

Anal fistulas commonly present as a recurrent perianal discharge. The external opening is often visible, the fistula track and the internal opening being palpable on digital examination. Fistulas can be classified into five groups according to their position relative to the anal sphincter. Treatment in all cases is surgical, and at its simplest consists of laying open and curetting the track, and leaving it to heal by secondary intention. Antibiotics are ineffective in the treatment of anal fistula.

Pruritus ani

Anal itching is a common symptom requiring careful evaluation. The commoner causes include:
• poor hygiene;
• anal pathology—haemorrhoids, fissure, fistula;
• infections—particularly fungal and parasitic;
• dermatological—eczema, atrophic dermatoses;
• drug reactions—contact sensitivities; and
• dietary excesses, e.g., coffee, chocolate.
    General treatment measures include careful washing of the area with water only, gentle but thorough drying, avoidance of scratching and avoidance of topical preparations.

Perianal warts

Condylomata acuminata are caused by infection with human papillomavirus. Treatment options include chemical methods (podophyllin), electrocautery or diathermy. Simple scissor excision is effective in 75% of cases.

11

Proctalgia fugax

Characterized by intense nocturnal pain in the anus and perineum which wakes the sufferer, the cause of proctalgia fugax is uncertain. Attacks are of limited duration and may be eased by simple analgesics. Quinine bisulphate, amyl nitrite and inhaled salbutamol have also been used with benefit.

References

1 Nelson R, Wagget J, Lennard-Jones JE, Barnes PRH. Constipation and megacolon in children and adults. In: Misiewicz JJ, Pounder RE, Venables CW. *Diseases of the Gut and Pancreas*, 2nd edn. Oxford: Blackwell Scientific Publications, 1994.

2 American Psychiatric Association. *Diagnostic and Statistical Manual of Mental Disorders*, 4th edn. Washington, DC: American Psychiatric Association, 1994.

3 Loening-Baucke V. Chronic constipation in children. *Gastroenterology* 1993; **105**: 1557–63.

4 RCR Working Party. *Making the Best Use of a Department of Clinical Radiology: Guidelines for Doctors*, 4th edn. London: The Royal College of Radiologists, 1998.

5 Pitzalis G, Mariani P, Chiarini-Testa MR *et al.* Lactitol in chronic idiopathic constipation of childhood. *Pediatr Med Chirur* 1995; **17**: 223–6.

6 Mooren GCAH, Van der Plas RN, Bossuyt PMM, Taminiau JAJM, Buller HA. The connection between dietary fibre intake and chronic constipation in children. *Ned Tijdschr Geneeskd* 1996; **140**: 2036–9.

7 Van der Plas RN, Benninga MA, Buller HA *et al.* Biofeedback training in treatment of childhood constipation: a randomised controlled study. *Lancet* 1996; **348**: 776–80.

8 Loening-Baucke V. Biofeedback treatment for chronic constipation and encopresis in childhood: long term outcome. *Paediatrics* 1995; **96**: 105–10.

9 Petticrew M, Watt I, Sheldon T. Systematic review of the effectiveness of laxatives in the elderly. *Health Technol Assessment (South Hampton, NY)* 1997; **1** (13): i–iv, 1–52.

10 Farthing MJG. Traveller's diarrhoea: mechanisms, manifestations and management. *Medicine* 1998; **26** (8): 33–9.

11 Ahmed SK, Thompson HJ. The effect of breakfast on minor anal complaints; a matched case-control study. *J R Coll Surg Edinb* 1997; **42** (5): 331–3.

12 Perez-Miranda M, Gomez-Cedenilla A, Leon-Colombo T, Pajares J, Mate-Jimenez J. Effect of fiber supplements on internal bleeding. *Hepato-gastroenterology* 1996; **43** (12): 1504–7.

13 McCrae HM, McLeod RS. Comparison of haemorrhoidal treatments: a meta-analysis. *Can J Surg* 1997; **40** (1): 14–17.

14 Lund JN, Scholefield JH. A randomised, prospective, double-blind, placebo-controlled trial of glyceryl trinitrate ointment in treatment of anal fissure. *Lancet* 1997; **349**: 11–14.

11

12 Colorectal cancer

Rob Wilson

Key Points

- A GP sees one or two new cases of colorectal cancer per year.
- Overall 5-year survival rate is less than 40%.
- Presenting symptoms include rectal bleeding, alteration in bowel habit and abdominal pain.
- Treatment is surgical excision, combined with adjuvant chemotherapy for Dukes' C lesions, plus adjuvant radiotherapy for Dukes' C rectal carcinoma.

Risk factors

These include genetic and environmental factors as well as pre-existing disease and association with other conditions.

It is felt that 5–10% of colorectal cancer may have an underlying genetic aetiology (Table 12.1) [1]. Genetic conditions associated with the development of polyps give an increased risk of colorectal cancer. Most has perhaps been written about familial adenomatous polyposis but hereditary non-polyposis colorectal cancer (HNPCC) is now much more readily recognized [2]. This covers site-specific colon cancer (Lynch type one) where two-thirds of the tumours are in the right side of the colon and also cancer family syndrome (Lynch type two) where, in addition to bowel cancer, there is a propensity to other gastrointestinal cancers as well as ovarian, uterine and renal tumours.

Environmental factors involved are still a matter of debate but pre-existing disease is certainly thought to give increased risk of colorectal cancer. This includes ulcerative colitis in which risk increases depending on a younger age of onset and, although Crohn's disease was felt to be associated with less risk of bowel cancer than ulcerative colitis, this has recently been disputed [3].

Table 12.1 Life-time risk of developing colorectal cancer [9].

> Population risk 1 : 50
> First-degree relative over 45 affected: risk 1 : 17
> First-degree relative and one second-degree relative affected: risk 1 : 12
> First-degree relative under 45 affected: risk 1 : 10
> Two first-degree relatives affected: risk 1 : 6
> More than two first-degree relatives affected: risk 1 : 2

Pathology

It is generally believed that most tumours follow the adenoma carcinoma sequence and begin as polyps [4]. Adenomas coexist with cancers in one-third of cases and 98% of colorectal carcinomas are adenocarcinomas. The risk of a polyp becoming malignant increases with size and polyps over 2 cm (up to 20%) have a 46% chance of becoming malignant. This also depends on histological type so that hyperplastic polyps carry no risk, tubular adenomas 5% risk, tubulovillous 22% risk and villous 40% risk. Despite many attempts to improve on Dukes' original classification for staging for bowel cancer [5], this has not yet been achieved. Dukes suggested that in stage A the disease was limited to the mucosa, in B it involved the muscularis mucosae, and in C it spread to regional lymph nodes. A fourth stage, Dukes' D, where spread includes metastases to other organs [6], is now generally accepted.

The extent of the problem

In 1996 there were over 28 000 new cases of colorectal cancer diagnosed in the UK and in the same year large bowel cancer was responsible for over 15 000 deaths in England and Wales [7]. It is the second most common cause of cancer death after lung cancer. Over 20% of patients present with metastases and the overall 5-year survival rate is less than 40% [8].

The incidence ratio for males to females is 1.3 : 1 for colonic and 1.5 : 1 for rectal tumours [10]. The peak incidence is in the 60- to 75-year age group.

Presentation and symptoms

Common symptoms include change of bowel habit, lower abdominal

12

colicky pains and rectal bleeding. Anorexia and weight loss are usually signs of more advanced disease. Many patients have few or no symptoms. Rectal bleeding is of course an important finding. In a 10-year study looking at 'walk-in' clinics in the USA of 201 individuals reporting rectal bleeding, 24% had serious disease of whom 13% overall had polyps and 6.5% colon cancer. It was concluded that when rectal bleeding is present investigations, including visualization of the entire colon, are important [11]. Some studies suggest that bleeding is rare if a tumour is proximal to the splenic flexure.

Colorectal cancer is highly unlikely (less than 1% of patients) in those who see blood only on toilet paper [12]. This study found three variables to be significantly predictive of cancer: (i) age; (ii) change in bowel habit; and (iii) blood on or mixed with the stool [12]. A study by questionnaire of people over the age of 50 in the north-east of England showed that 12% had experienced rectal bleeding, of whom half saw their doctor because of it [13]. This study also demonstrated delay in presentation due to a belief that the symptom was unlikely to be serious.

Delay between onset of symptoms and treatment is common, with a median of around 10 months [14]. Delay in presenting to the GP was even longer and on average people waited 3 years before consulting [13]. Whereas it is logical to assume that earlier treatment leads to better prognosis, this matter is still very much in the balance, with some studies showing such a relationship and others not [15]. It is often the case that bleeding may be due to haemorrhoids but inadequate investigation, notably of anaemia, can certainly add to the delay [16].

Other symptoms are, however, important and these include abdominal pain, anorexia, weight loss, tenesmus and mucorrhoea.

Clinical diagnosis and investigations

The key to success in investigations is to examine the whole of the large bowel. This can be done either by colonoscopy or by sigmoidoscopy plus double-contrast barium enema. Studies have shown these to have similar diagnostic yields and costs, but this depends on the expertise of the investigator [17]. Preoperative staging with at least liver ultrasound is also recommended to detect potential metastases.

Management

Management should be according to a series of well-accepted

guidelines [15,18–20]. Surgery is the first line of treatment, the outcome depending on case mix and surgeon grade. Survival can vary tremendously from surgeon to surgeon even when other variables are controlled [21]. In some studies no volume or specialization effects were found, but others have found that for a variety of reasons patients treated in larger hospitals or oncology centres have better survival. Under any circumstances it is known that long-term survival can occur only when the tumour has been completely removed.

The value of Dukes' staging [5] is in its prediction of prognosis with general figures suggesting 5-year survival rates of 90%, 45% and 25% in Dukes' stages A, B and C [22]. Initial studies focused on the clearance of the tumour up and down the bowel, but later studies concentrated on obtaining a healthy circumferential margin of tissue. The most recent studies have further concentrated on ensuring that the mesorectum leading up to the colon is properly cleared in an operation known as total mesorectal excision. This is thought to reduce recurrence rates and improve survival [23]. Surgery in the lower part of the bowel is aimed at preserving the sphincteric mechanism and avoiding a permanent stoma. When the tumour is very low rectal, this may be impossible and abdominoperineal resection is unavoidable.

Approximately 15% of patients present as emergencies with either obstruction of the bowel or perforation. The results in these cases are worse with a higher incidence of stomas.

Adjuvant therapy in most cases is given postoperatively. For patients with Dukes' C carcinoma, chemotherapy is used for colon cancer and chemotherapy and radiotherapy for rectal cancer. Postoperative patients with Dukes' B tumours are still treated on a trial basis. Preoperative radiotherapy has until now been confined to patients with fixed rectal cancers but a new MRC study is just under way, evaluating the effect of preoperative radiotherapy for mobile rectal carcinomas. Survival of patients with advanced or recurrent colorectal disease can be improved with chemotherapy, but only marginally, and the usual balance between survival and quality of life needs to be made on an individual case basis.

12

Improving care

The Effective Healthcare Bulletin [20] released by the NHS Centre for Reviews and Dissemination at the University of York suggests a series of key areas to improve quality of care (Table 12.2).

Table 12.2 Management of colorectal cancer.

---

1 *Patient focus*
The need for full verbal and written information about the patient's condition is generic to all cancer work but nowhere more pertinent than in colorectal cancer

2 *Multi-disciplinary teams*
A team working to agreed protocols and guidelines should form a core part of cancer care. This should include clinicians of mixed expertise, specialist nursing staff, professions allied to medicine and support and advisory services

3 *Endoscopy/radiology*
Adequate facilities for full visualization of the colon are essential

4 *Surgery for rectal cancer*
Surgery should be performed by a core of individuals with established expertise who are open to critical appraisal of their results with regard to curative resection rates, local recurrence rates and overall survival

5 *Improved pathology reporting*
Pathology reporting should be comprehensive and standardized with an agreed minimum data set on the basis of the Royal College of Surgeons and Association of Coloproctologists' Guidelines [18]

6 *Other treatments*
Preoperative radiotherapy should be available when indicated. Adjuvant chemotherapy can be useful under given circumstances and all case histories should be discussed in multi-disciplinary team meetings

7 *Follow-up*
Routine intensive follow-up does not seem to make a large difference to patient survival, but patients themselves often seem to prefer some contact with the hospital

---

References

1 Macklin MT. Inheritance of cancer of the stomach and large intestine in men. *J Watt Cancer Inst* 1960; **24**: 551–71.
2 Lynch HT. Genetics, natural history, tumour spectrum and pathology of hereditary non polyposis colorectal cancer. An updated review. *Dis Colon Rectum* 1993; **104**: 1535–49.
3 Lightdale CJ, Stemberg SS, Posner G. Carcinoma complicating Crohn's disease. *Am J Med* 1975; **59** (2): 262–8.
4 Morson BC. A polyp cancer sequence in the large bowel. *Proc R Soc Med* 1974; **67**: 451.

12

5 Dukes CE. The classification of cancer of the rectum. *Br J Surg* 1929; **17**: 643–8.
6 Turnbull RB, Kyle K, Watson FR, Spratt J. Cancer of the colon: the influence of no-touch isolation survival rates. *Ann Surg* 1967; **166**: 420–7.
7 Office of National Statistics. *Monitor*. London: HMSO, 1997.
8 Cancer Research Campaign. *Facts on Cancer*. Fact Sheets 18.1–18.4, 1993.
9 Lovett E. Family studies in cancers of the colon and rectum. *Br J Surg* 1976; **63**: 13–18.
10 Fraser P, Adelstein AM. Colorectal cancer—recent trends. *Recent Results Cancer Res* 1982; **83**: 1–10.
11 Helford M, Morton K, Zimmer-Gembeck M, Sox H. History of visible rectal bleeding in a primary care population. *JAMA* 1997; **277**: 44–8.
12 Fitjen G, Starmons R, Muris J, Shouten H, Blifham G, Knottnerus J. Preductive value of signs and symptoms for colorectal cancer in patients with rectal bleeding in general practice. *Family Prac* 1995; **12**: 279–86.
13 Crosland A, Jones R. Rectal bleeding: prevalence and consultation behaviour. *BMJ* 1995; **311**: 486–8.
14 Holliday H, Hardcastle J. Delay in diagnosis and treatment of symptomatic colorectal cancer. *Lancet* 1979; **i**: 309–11.
15 NHS. *Improving Outcomes in Colorectal Cancer. The Research Evidence*. London: NHS Executive, 1997.
16 Stebbling J, Nash A. Avoidable delay in management of carcinoma of the right colon. *Ann R Coll Surg Engl* 1995; **77**: 21–3.
17 Rex DK, Weddle RA, Lehman GA *et al.* Flexible sigmoidoscopy plus air contrast barium enema versus colonoscopy for suspected lower gastrointestinal bleeding. *Gastroenterology* 1990; **98**: 855–61.
18 *Guidelines for the Management of Colorectal Cancer*. London: Royal College of Surgeons of England and Association of Coloproctology, 1997.
19 *NHS Guidance on Commissioning Cancer Services. Improving Outcome in Colorectal Cancer*. The Manual. London: NHS Executive, 1997.
20 The Management of Colorectal Cancer. *Effective Health Care* 1997; **3** (6): 1–12.
21 McArdle CS, Hole D. Impact of variability among surgeons on postoperative morbidity and mortality and ultimate survival. *BMJ* 1991; **302**: 1501–5.
22 Goligher JC. *Surgery of the Anus, Rectum and Colon*, 4th edn. London: Ballière Tindall, 1980: 375.
23 MacFarlane JK, Ryall RDH, Heald RJ. Mesorectal excision for rectal cancer. *Lancet* 1993; **341**: 457–60.

12

Index

Page references to tables appear in **bold** type

access to care 4–5
acid reflux *see* gastro-oesophageal reflux
acid suppressants
    dyspepsia 31
    gastro-oesophageal reflux 16–17
    H_2-receptor blockers 16, 31
    proton pump inhibitors 16–17, 31
alcohol
    and acid reflux 14
    see also alcoholic liver disease
alcoholic liver disease 45, 47
    clinical diagnosis and investigations 49
    follow-up and prognosis 52
    management 52
    presentation and symptoms 48
alginates, in gastro-oesophageal reflux 14
ambulatory pH monitoring 13
5-aminosalicylic acid 86
amoxicillin, in acute cholecystitis 40
amyl nitrite, in proctalgia fugax 97
anaemia, and coeliac disease 76
anal conditions 95–7, **96**
anal fissures 95–6
anal fistula 97
analgesics
    acute cholecystitis 40
    haemorrhoids 96
    pancreatitis 59
    pethidine 40
antacids
    dyspepsia 30–1
    gastro-oesophageal reflux 14, 30
    side effects 31
anti-gliadin antibodies 78
anti-inflammatory drugs
    corticosteroids 51
    mesalazine 87
    NSAIDs 9, 23, 24
    sulphasalazine 87
anti-virals
    interferon alfa 52
    lamivudine 52
    ribavirin 52
antibiotics
    amoxicillin 40
    cephalosporins 40
    clarithromycin 29–30
antinuclear factor 47
aspirin
    and dyspepsia 24
    and gastro-oesophageal reflux 9
autoimmune hepatitis *see* autoimmune liver
    disease

autoimmune liver disease 46, 47
    clinical diagnosis and investigations 49–50
    management 51
    presentation and symptoms 48
azathioprine 87

barium meal 13, 35
Barrett's oesophagus 11–12
    management 18
beta-blockers
    ascites 52
    salbutamol 97
bile reflux 9–10
biliary colic 40, 41
bisacodyl **93**
bran **93**
budesonide 86
bulking agents **93**

Campylobacter 95
cephalosporins, in acute cholecystitis 40
chest pain, non-cardiac 10
children
    constipation in 91, 92
    Crohn's disease in 87–8
    diarrhoea in 94–5
    inflammatory bowel disease in 87–8
chocolate, and acid reflux 14
cholecystectomy 40–1
    laparoscopic 42
    open 42
    post-operative problems 41
cholecystitis
    acute 40
    chronic 40–1
chronic viral hepatitis 46, 48
    clinical diagnosis and investigations 50–2
    follow-up and prognosis 53
    management 52
    presentation and symptoms 49
cimetidine 16
cisapride 15, 18
clarithromycin 29–30
clinical management, rules of 3
CLO test 28
codeine phosphate 87
coeliac disease 73–9
    background 73–4
    clinical diagnosis and investigations 75–7
    complications of 76–7, **77**
    conditions associated with 75–7
        anaemia 76
        dermatitis herpetiformis 75

Down's syndrome 75–6
  insulin-dependent diabetes 75
  malignancy 77
  metabolic bone disease 76
follow-up and prognosis 77
incidence 74
presentation and common symptoms 74
screening and prevention 78
useful resources 78–9
coffee, and acid reflux 14
colorectal cancer 99–104
  clinical diagnosis and investigations 101
  incidence 100
  management 101–3, **103**
  pathology 100
  presentation and symptoms 100–1
  risk factors 99–100, **100**
common bile duct stones 41
computed tomography, of pancreas 58
condylomata acuminata 97
constipation 91–4
  adult 92
  childhood 92
  diagnosis 92
  and haemorrhoids 95–6
  intervention options 93–4
  outcome measures 92–3
  prevalence 91
  prognosis 94
corticosteroids, in autoimmune liver disease 51
cost effectiveness 4–5
Crohn's disease *see* inflammatory bowel disease
Crosby Capsule 75

danthron **93**
dapsone, in dermatitis herpetiformis 75
dermatitis herpetiformis, and coeliac disease 75
diabetes, and coeliac disease 75
diagnostic acid suppression test 14
diarrhoea 94–5
  traveller's 95
diathermy 97
diet
  food intolerance 63–4
  and gastro-oesophageal reflux **10**
  gluten-free 73, 75, 76, 77
  and irritable bowel syndrome 63–4
diuretics, in ascites 52
docusate **93**
domperidone 15
Down's syndrome, and coeliac disease 75–6
Dukes' staging for colorectal cancer 100, 102
dyspepsia 23–32
  background 23–4, **24**
  causes **24**
  H. pylori eradication 26–8, **27**
  presentation and investigation 25–6, **25**

testing for *H. pylori* 28–9, **29**
  treatment 29–31
    acid suppressing drugs 31
    antacids 30–1
    H. pylori eradication therapy 29–30, **30**
dysphagia, in gastric cancer 34

electrocautery 97
encopresis 91
endomysial antibodies 78
cholangiopancreatography 40, 41, 58
Escherichia coli 95
evidence, definition of 2–3
evidence-based medicine 1–8
  background 1–2
  cost reduction and access to care 4–5
  definition of evidence 2–3
  imposition of management rules 3
  new skills 3–4
  objections to 4
  practice of 5–6, **5**
extra-corporeal shock wave lithotripsy 42

faecal softeners **93**
food intolerance 63–4

gallbladder 39–43
  biliary colic 40, 41
  cholecystectomy 40–1, 42
    post-operative problems 41
  cholecystitis 40–1
  common bile duct stones 41
  gallstones 39, 41
    medical management 42
    silent 41
gallstones 40
  cholesterol stones 39
  medical management 42
  pigment stones 39
  silent 41
  see also gallbladder
gas bloat syndrome 17
gastric cancer 33–8
  clinical diagnosis and investigations 34–5
  follow-up and prognosis 36
  incidence 34
  management 35–6
  presentation, diagnosis and investigation 34
  screening and prevention 36
  staging 35
gastric freezing 2–3
gastro-oesophageal reflux 9–21
  causes of 9–10, **10**
  clinical diagnosis and investigations 12–14
  foods associated with **10**
  incidence 10–11
  management 14–19
    acid suppression drugs 16–17
    antacids and alginates 14
    Barrett's oesophagus 18

lifestyle measures 14
long-term therapy 18
motility-altering drugs 15
mucosal protection therapy 15
'step-up' or 'step-down' therapy **19**
surgical management 17
presentation and common symptoms
11–12
gastroscopy 13
gluten-free diet 73, 75, 76, 77
glycerol **93**

H$_2$-receptor blockers 16, 31
cimetidine 16
dyspepsia 31
gastric cancer 35
nizatidine 16
ranitidine 15, 16, 18
haemorrhoids 95–6
Helicobacter pylori
and duodenal ulcer 24
eradication 26–8, **27**, 29–30, **30**
and gastric cancer 33
and gastro-oesophageal reflux 10
testing for 28–9, **29**
hepatitis, autoimmune *see* autoimmune liver
disease
hepatitis B *see* chronic viral hepatitis
hepatitis C *see* chronic viral hepatitis
hereditary non-polyposis colorectal cancer
99
hiatus hernia 9–10
hypolactasia, adult-acquired 63–4

immuno-modulating drugs
azothiaprine 87
6-mercaptopurine 87
inflammatory bowel disease 81–9
background 81
clinical diagnosis and investigations 83–4,
83
epidemiology and prevalence 82
management 85–8
in childhood 87–8
information sources 85–6
long-term management 87
referral 88
treatment 86–7
presentation and common symptoms 83
screening 84–5
interferon alfa 52
irritable bowel syndrome 61–71
clinical diagnosis and investigations 67
consultation rates 65–7
diet 63–4
epidemiology 64–5, **65**
management 67–9
mood and gastrointestinal function 61–2
post-infective 63
presentation and common symptoms
65–7

psychological abnormalities 62–3
visceral hypersensitivity 62
ispaghula husk **93**

lactose intolerance 63–4
lactulose **93**
lamivudine 52
lansoprazole 16, 19
laxatives 92–3, **93**
liver 45–55
alcoholic liver disease 45, 47
clinical diagnosis and investigations 49
follow-up and prognosis 52
management 52
presentation and symptoms 48
autoimmune liver disease 46, 47
clinical diagnosis and investigations
49–50
management 51
presentation and symptoms 48
chronic viral hepatitis 46, 48
clinical diagnosis and investigations
50–1
follow-up and prognosis 53
management 52
presentation and symptoms 49
primary biliary cirrhosis 46, 47
clinical diagnosis and investigations
50
follow-up and prognosis 53
management 51
presentation and symptoms 49
screening and prevention 53
loperamide 87
lymphoma, and coeliac disease 77

magnetic resonance
cholangiopancreatography 58
malabsorption *see* coeliac disease
6-mercaptopurine 87
mesalazine 87
metabolic bone disease, and coeliac disease
76
metoclopramide 15
metronidazole 30
mood, and gastrointestinal function 61–2
motility-altering drugs 15
cisapride 15, 17
domperidone 15
metoclopramide 15
mucosal protection therapy 15
sucralfate 15

National Association for Colitis and Crohn's
Disease 85–6, 88
Nissen fundoplication 17
nitroglycerin ointment 96
nizatidine 16
non-steroidal anti-inflammatory drugs
and dyspepsia 23, 24
and gastro-oesophageal reflux 9

non-ulcer dyspepsia 23–4
  see also dyspepsia

oesophageal manometry 13
oesophagitis 11
omeprazole 16, 29–30
oral contraception, and inflammatory bowel
      disease 82
oral hypoglycaemics, in pancreatitis 59
osmotic laxatives **93**
osteoporosis, in Crohn's disease 86–7

pancreatitis 57–60
  acute 57–8
    aetiology and presentation 57
    management 57–8
  chronic 58–9
    aetiology 58–9
    management 59
  pancreatic insufficiency 59
  pancreatic pain 59
paraffin **93**
peptic ulcer disease *see* dyspepsia
perianal warts 97
pethidine, in acute cholecystitis 40
podophyllin 97
polyethylene glycol **93**
prednisolone 86
  side effects 86–7
primary biliary cirrhosis 46, 47
  clinical diagnosis and investigations 50
  follow-up and prognosis 53
  management 51
  presentation and symptoms 49
proctalgia fugax 97
proton pump inhibitors 16–17, 18–19, 31
  dyspepsia 31
  H. pylori eradication 29–30

lansoprazole 16, 19
  omeprazole 16, 29–30
  potential problems 17
pruritus ani 97

quinine bisulphate, in proctalgia fugax
      97

ranitidine 15, 16, 18
ribavirin 52

salbutamol, in proctalgia fugax 97
senna **93**
Shigella 95
smoking
  and acid reflux 14
  and inflammatory bowel disease
      82
  and peptic ulcer 24
smooth muscle antibody 47
sodium pico-sulphate **93**
steatohepatitis 45
steatorrhoea 58
stenting, in gastric cancer 35
stimulant laxatives **93**
sucralfate 15
sulphapyridine, in dermatitis herpetiformis
      75
sulphasalazine 87

traveller's diarrhoea **95**

ulcerative colitis *see* inflammatory bowel
      disease
13C-urea breath test 28
ursodeoxycholic acid 51

visceral hypersensitivity 62